The Sweetener Book

by D. Eric Walters, Ph.D.

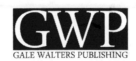

Gale Walters Publishing
Lindenhurst, Illinois

Gale Walters Publishing

1711 East Grand Avenue

Lindenhurst, Illinois 60046

www.galewalters.com

ISBN 978-0-9891092-0-8

Library of Congress Control Number: 2013904391

Cover photo: Valerie P. Anderson

Cover design: Paula E. Anderson

Edition 1.0

For updates, visit www.sweetenerbook.com

To my parents, Dave and Sally Walters.

Table of Contents

Preface

Why am I writing a book about sweeteners?

It needs to be done. Consumers now have over 20 choices of sweeteners. There is a lot of misinformation about these sweeteners in the media and on the web. Someone needs to sift through the thousands of scientific papers and regulatory agency publications, and put the real, bottom line information into a form that consumers can use.

Why me?

I believe I am qualified to do this for several reasons. First, I have a degree in Pharmacy and a Ph.D. in Medicinal Chemistry. I've learned how chemical substances interact with the human body. I've learned about metabolism, diabetes, and the ways that the human body handles xenobiotics (substances we encounter and consume in our environment).

I spent 12 years working in the food industry, at Kraft Foods and at the NutraSweet Company. I carried out research into the discovery of new sweeteners, and I looked in depth at the ways sweeteners work.

When I left industry in 1992, I became a professor at Rosalind Franklin University. I've spent the last 21 years there doing research and teaching in the College of Pharmacy, the Medical School, and the Graduate School. My current areas of research include sweeteners, antiviral drugs, and antibiotics. I also teach a course in communicating scientific information, and I've written a book on that subject (*Scientists Must Speak*, co-authored with my wife, Gale Walters, who is a food scientist). Conducting research and communicating science are my passions.

On several occasions I have been called on as an expert witness. The United States International Trade Commission, the United States Patent Office, and the U.S. District Court in Philadelphia have all recognized me as an expert in the chemistry and biology of sweeteners.

Disclaimers, claimers, and disclosures:
I am not a medical doctor, so you should not construe my opinions as medical advice. I am a scientist and a teacher, and I want you to know that my opinions are based on over 30 years of study. I've been in academia for the last 21 years, and I value my independence, so I don't feel that I am biased for or against my previous employers. I have occasionally consulted for a number of companies, dealing with many different sweeteners. None of those companies has paid me enough money to buy my objectivity. The opinions I offer here are exactly the same ones I offer to my diabetic father, who has a serious sweet tooth, and who I love dearly.

Acknowledgments:
I thank Valerie Anderson, Hope T. Bilyk, R.D., L.D.N., Mimi Daykin, R.D., C.D.N., Javier Lopez, Ph.D., Salli Peterson, R.D., Rick and Laurie Riggle, and Gale Walters for their critical reading and their suggestions for improvement of the manuscript.

Eric Walters, 2013

Introduction

Why is sweetness such a big deal?

Let's start at the beginning. Why are we wired to like sweet taste so much?

The basic tastes (sweet, bitter, salty, sour, umami and probably others) serve important purposes. Umami detects the presence of protein, an essential part of the daily diet. Salty taste detects sodium and chloride, important electrolytes. Sour taste can alert us to spoilage, and bitterness is associated with many toxic substances in our environment. Sweetness (up until the last 100 years) has almost always meant sugar, a signal for foods that contain usable energy.

For most of human existence, it would have been useful to associate pleasure and craving with sugar (and the calories that come with it). Only in the industrial age have we had so much access to sugar that sweetness from sugar represents a health problem.

The sweet taste receptors that detect sugars are rather unique, compared to other receptors. Receptors that detect hormones and neurotransmitters, for example, are exquisitely sensitive. They can respond to a millionth of a gram or less of the substance they are to detect. But a millionth of a gram of sugar would not provide enough energy for you to walk to the front door! So sweet taste receptors are, by comparison, very insensitive. They don't detect sweetness unless the stuff in your mouth is at least 1% sugar, and that's a low level of sweetness. Fresh fruits usually contain 5 to 12% sugar. Carbonated soft drinks and fruit juices are usually in the neighborhood of 10% sugar.

So the human body is hard-wired to enjoy sweetness, specifically sweetness corresponding to 5 to 10% sugar. It's easy to see why the combination of a sedentary lifestyle and easy access to sugar makes it easy (and even pleasant!) to consume far more calories than we need.

How taste works

"Taste" versus "Flavor"

What do we mean when we talk about "taste"? We are talking about what we sense on the tongue. "Flavor" is a broader term, that includes aromas. When you drink fresh orange juice, you have no problem identifying the orange flavor. You could detect it by smelling the juice before you ever put it in your mouth. Once it's in your mouth, the "orangeness" is even stronger, because the aromatic flavor molecules are warmed in your mouth and move retronasally (through the back of your mouth into your sinuses) to your olfactory (odor-detecting) tissues. In your mouth, your taste buds detect *sweetness* and *sourness*. Sweet and sour are tastes, and the "orangeness" is flavor.

The basic tastes

What can we taste? There are several basic tastes that we detect.

- *Sweet*. Table sugar (sucrose) has a clean sweet taste. Many other sugars taste sweet as well. And we have discovered a number of things other than sugars that taste sweet.
- *Salty*. Table salt (sodium chloride) is the standard reference for salty taste. Other salts may have some saltiness as well as other tastes. There aren't any really good salt substitutes yet.
- *Sour*. Anything acidic has sour taste. Vinegar has both sour taste and an acetic acid aroma (flavor). Citric acid (used in most sour candies) is just plain sour.
- *Bitter*. Caffeine, cocoa, and quinine are examples of bitter-tasting things we often consume. Bitterness is usually considered unpleasant, although many people like it in moderation or in combination with sweetness.
- *Umami*. "Umami" is a Japanese word that means "delicious". It is used to describe a savory, brothy taste. In most animals, the umami receptor is sensitive to many of the amino acids that make up proteins. In humans, it is mainly sensitive to a single amino acid, glutamate, that is present in all proteins. Glutamate and other amino acids are released when proteins begin to break down, through cooking (think of chicken broth) or through the activity of enzymes (aging cheese, or yeast extract). You can add it to your food as monosodium glutamate (MSG).
- *Fat*. There is growing evidence that we may have taste receptors to detect fat. We probably do not taste the more abundant triglyceride fat in our diet, but the free fatty acids that are released when triglycerides break down. What kinds of foods have these free fatty acids? French fries, as the cooking oil breaks down. Cheese, as the butterfat breaks down. Chocolate, as the cocoa butter is processed. We don't have a good descriptive word for fat taste yet, but it seems to be something that many of us like.
- *Calcium*. We may also be able to taste calcium as a distinct taste quality. Too much calcium produces a sensation of "chalkiness," which is not considered pleasant, but a low level of calcium may contribute to pleasant taste.

How sweet taste works

Look closely at your tongue in the mirror. The surface is quite rough. There are a lot of bumps sticking up. These are called *papillae* (a single one of them is called a *papilla*). These aren't the *taste buds*, but many of them *contain* taste buds.

There are four kinds of papillae.

- Across the back of the tongue (quite far back), there are several very large round circumvallate papillae. They are surrounded by a trough-like groove, and these grooves contain clusters of about 50 cells. These clusters of cells are taste buds. The actual taste buds are too small to see without a microscope.

- On both sides of the tongue, near the back, are the foliate papillae. They are also quite large, but they're so far back they may be difficult to see. They have several grooves or folds (that's where the name comes from), and these folds also contain taste buds.

- All over the surface of the tongue are the fungiform papillae. These are smaller, with a shape reminiscent of mushrooms (again, that's the source of the name). They have taste buds on their surface.

- Also all over the surface of the tongue are the filiform papillae. These are even smaller than the fungiform papillae, and they do not have taste buds.

Now let's take a close-up look at the taste buds. The cells are clustered together in a little ball, and the individual cells are fairly elongated. One end of the cluster is at the surface of the tongue, exposed to the saliva through a pore. This is the end that detects taste. At the opposite end, some of the cells are connected to nerve fibers that carry the taste signal to the brain.

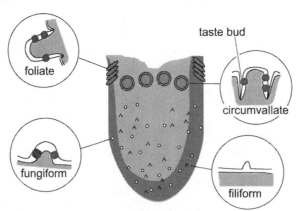

If we increase the magnification at the taste pore, we can see that some of the taste bud cells have *microvilli*, long thin parts that extend into the taste pore. These provide a lot of surface area for the *receptors*, structures on the taste cell surface that detect molecules responsible for taste. Receptors are sometimes compared to locks, and the molecules that fit into them are like keys. If the "key" fits into the "keyhole" on the "lock", then the cell sends a signal to the brain. Sweeteners are the keys that unlock the sweet receptors, bitter-tasting molecules are the keys that unlock the bitterness receptors, and so on. Saccharin, which tastes both sweet and bitter, can fit into both kinds of receptors.

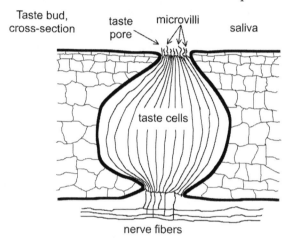

Taste bud, cross-section — taste pore — microvilli — saliva — taste cells — nerve fibers

What kinds of receptors are there? Since there are so many different kinds of sweeteners, it was once thought that there must be several different kinds of sweet taste receptors, but we now know there is a single kind of sweet taste receptor that recognizes all of the different substance we consider sweet. The sweet receptor is a large, complex molecule that provides several different "keyholes", so that different sweeteners can fit into different places.

In contrast, we have about 30 different kinds of bitterness receptors, so that we can recognize bitterness from many different sources. Interestingly, most people don't have the complete set, and different people are missing different ones. This accounts for individual differences in our perception of things that people may consider bitter. About half of the population detects a strong bitter taste in saccharin, and the other half does not. Some people detect a strong bitterness in vegetables such as broccoli, and others do not.

It has recently been discovered that there are sweet taste receptors in the intestine! We do not consciously sense the taste of the digesting food. The receptors are likely there to make sure the intestinal cells are prepared to absorb sugars when they are present. It has been suggested that artificial sweeteners might cause the intestine to become more efficient at absorbing sugars than it would otherwise be. It's also possible that these receptors might be involved in sending satiety signals to the brain.

How sweetness is measured

What does it mean when someone says that saccharin is 200 times as sweet as sugar? How is that measured?

Since sucrose is the most widely used sweetener, it has become the standard for measuring sweetness. A 1% solution of sucrose (1 gram of sucrose in 100 milliliters of water) is barely sweet. A soft drink is typically about 10% sucrose and tastes very sweet. Sweetness is usually measured using a panel of 10-15 trained humans. It is convenient for the panelists to use a 15 centimeter line scale, with anchor points at 0, 5, 10, and 15 centimeters. They practice with solutions of sucrose ranging from 1% to 15%, learning to mark a 5% solution near the 5 centimeter mark, an 8% solution at about 8 centimeters, and so forth. Then they are tested, using coded samples, to see how accurate they are. A well trained panel can provide good accuracy and precision (plus or minus 1 unit) in measuring sweetness this way.

Once the panel can provide good accuracy, the relative sweetness of other sweeteners can be determined. What concentration of saccharin will match the sweetness of 2% sucrose? It turns out that a 0.004% solution of saccharin is as sweet as 2% sucrose. That means that saccharin is about 500 times (2 divided by 0.004) as sweet as sucrose. A funny thing happens with high potency sweeteners, though. If we try to match 5% sucrose, it is only about 400 times as sweet. If we want to match 8% sucrose, saccharin comes out to about 200 times as sweet. So the sweetness potency isn't as high when we try to match higher sucrose levels. It starts to level out.

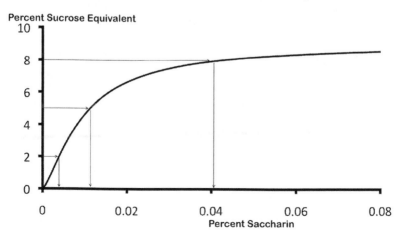

Saccharin Concentration vs Response

The sweetness potency also depends on what else is in the food or beverage. Some ingredients enhance sweetness, and others mask it, so food scientists who are designing a new product must adjust the amount of sweetener to get it just right for a particular product. It has also been found that better sweet taste quality is often possible if you use a combination of sweeteners. Each sweetener has its own characteristic off tastes. When you use a blend, the sweetness is additive or even synergistic, while the different off tastes stay at low levels.

How safety is assessed

First and foremost, please recognize that safety assessment is intended to be applicable for whole populations. Is this sweetener safe for the 300 million people who live in the United States? But each person is unique, so your result may vary. If sweetener X gives you a headache, don't use sweetener X! It may be that you have a unique combination of genetics and physiology that causes you to suffer an adverse effect. Or it may be some other ingredient that often accompanies that sweetener. Whatever the case, if any particular food ingredient causes you problems, it's best to avoid those problems.

You should be aware that adverse effects are sometimes caused by sweeteners (see the section on sugar alcohols, for example), and sometimes by other (often unidentified) factors. When aspartame was approved in the 1980s, the FDA monitored consumer complaints, and the most common complaint was headache. Many other reported complaints were very likely caffeine-related. A group of scientists at Duke University found 40 people who reported headaches from aspartame, who were willing to take part in a double-blind, placebo-controlled study (samples were coded, so neither the subject nor the experimenter knew when the subject received aspartame, and when he or she received placebo) [1]. Subjects received 30 milligrams per kilogram of aspartame (this corresponds to 11 cans of diet cola for a 150 pound person, 15 cans for a 200 pound person) or a placebo. The incidence of headache was 35% with aspartame, and 40% with placebo. The difference was not statistically significant. Either these people were simply prone to get headaches, or something else in their diet caused them headaches.

The sixteenth century Swiss physician Paracelsus recognized that everything is toxic, depending on the dose. Selenium is a good example. It's a micronutrient (the human body contains 20 mg or less) that is needed for several enzymes involved in processing thyroid hormones. However, consumption of 1 mg or more per day can lead to a condition called selenosis, which can be fatal. We see the same thing with some sweeteners. For example, glycyrrhizin, the sweet substance in licorice, can have beneficial anti-inflammatory effects. Glycyrrhizin inhibits the body's ability to break down cortisol, so more cortisol accumulates, and cortisol has anti-inflammatory effects. But too much licorice can lead to too much cortisol. Cortisol can cause fluid retention, which will have serious consequences for people with high blood pressure or kidney problems. Just because something is natural, that doesn't mean it is safe. Remember, cholera toxin is very natural, and very deadly.

Regulatory agencies

Until the end of the 19th century, adulteration and misbranding of foods was not well regulated. All sorts of artificial colors, some toxic, were sometimes added to foods. Saccharin could be used in place of sugar. Toxic substances could be used as preservatives. All of this could be done without any kind of labeling.

The Wiley Act, in 1906, led to the establishment of the FDA in the United States. The FDA and other regulatory agencies have established procedures to regulate what can be added to food, and how much can be added. In the United States, the 1958 Food, Drug & Cosmetic Act established rules for establishing the safety of "food additives" prior to their use in foods.

In the European Union, food additives are regulated by the European Food Safety Authority (EFSA). The European Union assigns identification numbers ("E-numbers") to all food additives, including sweeteners. For example, saccharin is E954, and sorbitol is E420.

Internationally, the Joint FAO/WHO Expert Committee on Food Additives (JECFA) assesses the safety of food additives. In Japan, food additives are regulated by the Ministry of Health, Labor and Welfare.

In the United States, in order to obtain regulatory approval for a new food additive (including sweeteners), the manufacturer must carry out extensive safety testing. These studies must include short-term tests for genetic toxicity, metabolism and pharmacokinetic studies, short-term toxicity tests in rodents, 90 day toxicity tests in rodents and in non-rodents, reproduction studies in animals, one year toxicity in non-rodents, and lifetime toxicity and carcinogenicity studies in rodents [2]. These are followed by clinical studies in humans.

The requirements for approval for a new food additive are more stringent than those for approval for a new drug. In the case of a drug, some level of adverse effects may be tolerated if the disease is worse than the adverse effects, or if no other treatment is available. But a food additive is likely to be consumed by large segments of the population, and no adverse effect is tolerable. This realization led to the establishment of the Acceptable Daily Intake.

Acceptable Daily Intake (ADI)

Safety testing must establish a level at which there is no observable adverse effect even with daily use. This level is called the "no observable adverse effect level (NOAEL). Regulatory agencies then set an Acceptable Daily Intake level (ADI) that is usually 1% of the NOAEL, to provide a 100-fold safety factor. The ADI is frequently expressed in terms of the number of milligrams per kilogram of body weight per day. To determine how many cans of diet soft drink you can consume per day, you need to know your weight (in kilograms), and the amount of sweetener used per can. For example, let's consider a 170 pound person (77 kilograms) drinking a diet cola with 180 milligrams of aspartame per can. The ADI for aspartame in the United States is 50 milligrams per kilogram per day, so our subject can consume 3,850 milligrams of aspartame per day (50 x 77). To get 3,850 milligrams of aspartame, this person would need to drink 21 cans of diet cola. And at that point, this person would have consumed *one one-hundredth* of the amount which *might* cause an adverse effect of any kind.

Following regulatory approval, the FDA often requires post-approval surveillance for new food additives. Aspartame, for example, underwent 8 years of post-approval surveillance following its approval in the early 1980s.

The GRAS exemption

When the 1958 law was passed, it was obviously impractical to go back and test the safety of every existing food additive, and it would have been a waste of resources to do so for things that everyone already knows to be safe. Therefore, the law created the "GRAS exemption," where "GRAS" is an acronym for "generally recognized as safe." In order to qualify for GRAS status, there must be general consensus among qualified experts that a food additive is safe, based on widely available information. This usually includes published, peer-reviewed safety studies, or evidence that a substance has been consumed safely for hundreds or thousands of years. The GRAS process has been used, for example, in the case of rebaudioside and other stevia-based sweeteners. In order for a food additive to achieve GRAS status, someone (usually a manufacturer) must file a GRAS notification with the FDA. The FDA publishes all such notifications, and anyone interested may comment. After a period of time, the FDA may accept or reject the additive, or it may request further data. The Flavor and Extract Manufacturers Association (FEMA) is a U.S. trade group that has an expert panel which reviews some ingredients and periodically publishes a list of substances that it considers GRAS. These substances are assigned FEMA GRAS numbers. For example, neohesperidin dihydrochalcone is FEMA GRAS 3811.

The internet abounds with conspiracy theories about one sweetener or another gaining regulatory approval in nefarious ways. But the reality is that there are many regulatory agencies all over the world evaluating the safety data for each sweetener. These agencies are generally run by risk-averse bureaucrats and highly skilled scientists. The history books contain a number of sweeteners (dulcin and P-4000, to name two) that were found to be unsafe and were discarded. Those sweeteners that have achieved regulatory approval around the world are, with a high degree of certainty, safe.

Calories, Glycemic Index, and Glycemic Load

Two of the most prevalent health issues we face are obesity and diabetes. Both of these drive people to use sweeteners other than sugar. There are two major reasons that people use sweeteners other than table sugar. One is to avoid the calories that come from sugars. The other is to avoid rapid increases in blood glucose levels.

With respect to calories, the sugars usually provide 4 calories per gram. That doesn't sound like a lot, until you realize that a 12 ounce soft drink has about 40 grams of sugar. If you usually drink several cans per day, switching to a no-calorie beverage could save you hundreds of calories per day. Note, I am not advocating that anyone should consume several cans of any soft drink, sugared or not, per day!

When people with diabetes talk about "blood sugar," they are concerned with the concentration of glucose in the blood. Glucose is the preferred energy source for the brain, and it is an important energy source in other organs as well. But an excessive level of glucose in the blood can lead to tissue damage. Normally, insulin can control the level of glucose in the blood, but for people with diabetes, the glucose concentration may be poorly regulated. People with diabetes need glucose, just like everyone else, but they must monitor their blood glucose level to ensure that the blood level stays within normal limits. If a person with diabetes consumes a lot of pure glucose, it may be absorbed rapidly, leading to an unsafe blood level. Starches and some sugars contain glucose, and they may release it rapidly or slowly. Other carbohydrates (and some of the sugar alcohols) may be converted to glucose, also at varying rates.

The *glycemic index* (GI) is a measure of how much a food increases blood glucose, relative to glucose itself, which is set to a value of 100. It's important to note that there are two different methods for measuring GI. One is based on a comparison to white bread, and the other is based on comparison to glucose. People generally agree that the comparison to glucose makes more sense, but you will still see values based on white bread, and often values you find on the web do not tell you which standard was used. I am using only the glucose-based scale in this book.

Measurement of the GI usually involves asking a group of human volunteers to consume 25 or 50 grams of glucose or the test material. Blood glucose is then measured several times over the next three hours, to determine how much the blood level changed. A comprehensive table of measured GI values for foods has been published [3].

Maltose (two glucose molecules linked together), maltodextrin (3-20 glucose molecules linked together in chains), and starch (chains of hundreds of glucose molecules) can all easily be digested, releasing glucose. Maltose and maltodextrin have a GI of 105, because they are rapidly converted to glucose, and on a weight basis, 100 grams of maltose can produce 105 grams of glucose. 100 grams of maltodextrin with chain length of 20 can produce 111 grams of glucose. Starches may have much lower GI values, depending on how readily the starch can be digested.

It's not enough to look at the glycemic index. Which is worse for the blood glucose level of a person with diabetes: a big plate of pasta, with a GI of 45, or a packet of artificial sweetener that contains a gram of maltodextrin, with GI of 105? Now we must talk about glycemic load (GL). This is a measure of the total amount of glucose that will enter the body. One unit of GL is approximately equivalent to consuming one gram of glucose, so 100 grams of glucose will have a GL of 100. Glycemic load is calculated by multiplying the GI of a food by the number of grams of carbohydrate in the food, then dividing by 100 (because GI is based on 100 grams of glucose, and GL is on a per-gram-of-glucose scale). In our example, a cup of cooked pasta with 40 grams of carbohydrates and a GI of 45 will have a GL of 18 (45 x 40 ÷ 100), and the packet of sweetener will have a GL of 1 (105 x 1 ÷ 100). The pasta, with 18 grams of glucose, provides a lot more glucose than the packet of sweetener, with 1 gram. People with diabetes, or anyone concerned about glucose, can use the glycemic load to monitor their glucose intake.

Carbohydrate requirements

The Institute of Medicine (IOM) is a non-profit organization established in 1970 by the National Academy of Sciences, which was chartered by President Lincoln in 1863. The goal of the IOM is "to provide unbiased and authoritative advice to decision makers and the public." The IOM points out that the brain is the only carbohydrate-dependent organ in the body. All of the others can get the energy they need by burning fat or protein if necessary. The IOM established a Recommended Dietary Intake (RDI) of 130 grams per day of carbohydrate for adults and children. This number is based on the amount of glucose used by the brain and is intended to be the minimum amount that is sufficient for the nutritional needs of most people. In reality, it is possible to survive without consuming carbohydrates, providing that the diet includes enough protein or fat so that the body can convert some of the amino acids (from the protein) or glycerol (from the fat) to glucose.

The IOM also recommends that added sugars should not exceed 25% of total energy intake. "Added sugars" refers to sugars that are added to foods or beverages that provide little or no vitamins, minerals, or other essential nutrients. Soft drinks, fruit drinks, desserts and candies are major sources of added sugars. The bottom line message is to consume carbohydrates in moderation.

Sweeteners, insulin, and appetite

Do sweeteners affect insulin levels? In general, we expect sweeteners that produce glucose to have an effect on insulin, and it is generally proportional to the glycemic index of the sweetener. This isn't at all surprising.

What about the sweeteners that have a zero glycemic index? Does the sensation of sweetness cause the body to release insulin? There have been dozens of experimental studies to try to answer this question. The experiments have been done in lab animals and in humans. They have been done with both normal and diabetic subjects. They have been done in both fasting and fed subjects. Occasionally, a small measurable effect on insulin is observed, but most of the studies do not show a significant effect of sweeteners on insulin.

Do artificial sweeteners have an effect on appetite or satiety? Appetite and satiety are rather subjective, and are difficult to measure in any quantitative way. In general, studies indicate that non-caloric sweeteners do not significantly affect appetite and satiety, either positively or negatively.

Do artificial sweeteners cause you to crave more sweets? Will artificial sweeteners help to control weight? Again, there have been dozens of studies. Sometimes, the results are not very clear-cut, especially in human subjects. It's very difficult to do such studies in humans and fully control dietary intake. And humans sometimes rationalize high calorie food choices by saying "It's okay. I had a diet soft drink with it." The Academy of Nutrition and Dietetics (formerly the American Dietetic Association) reviewed the literature and concluded [4] that many non-caloric sweeteners, "...as part of a comprehensive weight loss or maintenance program by individuals may be associated with greater weight loss and may assist individuals with weight maintenance over time." If using a low calorie sweetener helps you to consume fewer calories, it can probably help you to control weight. On the other hand, if you use a low calorie sweetener but do not lower your caloric intake, it will not help at all. Your own experience with this experiment is probably much more meaningful for you than any study that was done with rats or mice or college student volunteers.

Sweeteners and children

Which sweeteners are safe for children? Let's start with sugars. Sugars are certainly safe, in moderation. As described in a previous section, the Institute of Medicine has established a recommended minimum of 130 grams of carbohydrate (which includes sugars) per day, for normal brain function. The main problems with sugars are (1) that some children consume too much sugar, which can lead to obesity if too many calories are consumed, and (2) sugars can contribute to dental caries. It is very easy to exceed the recommended intake of sugars, since a can of sugar sweetened soft drink contains 39 grams of sugar, and a serving of fruit punch or grape juice may have even more. Moderation is really important.

Sugar alcohols are used extensively in "sugar-free" candy and in "no sugar added" ice creams. These are also are safe, in moderation. In this case, the main problem is that overconsumption can cause gastrointestinal problems (gas and a laxative effect). In the section on polyols, you'll find a table that lists "laxative threshold values." The values listed are for an adult. It is likely that these values will vary with body weight, so a small child is likely to be affected by a smaller quantity than the amount listed.

The high potency sweeteners, which have gone through regulatory approval, are considered safe for children. The FDA, for example, assumes that children will be consuming a food additive when the agency reviews the food additive petition. The Acceptable Daily Intake is established with all possible consumers, including children, in mind. It is inconceivable that a food additive which could harm children would be approved for use by adults.

Sweeteners and pregnancy and lactation

Which sweeteners are safe in pregnancy and for lactating women? Some women experience gestational diabetes while pregnant. This is a situation in which the body does not respond fully to insulin, and the blood's glucose level is higher than normal. If that happens, you should talk to your physician or dietitian about limiting your intake of sugars.

Sorbitol and the other sugar alcohols are considered to be safe during pregnancy. Keep in mind that these sweeteners, if consumed in excess, can cause gas and diarrhea. An extended bout of diarrhea could cause dehydration, which could be a cause for concern.

High potency sweeteners are approved for use during pregnancy and lactation. The Academy of Nutrition and Dietetics, in its Position Paper on the use of nutritive and nonnutrititve sweeteners, points out that regulatory approval of food additives requires multigenerational feeding studies in animals, in order to identify any possible risk to fetus or mother. As they point out, any nonnutritive sweetener found to be unsafe at any stage of life would not be approved for use [4].

Sweeteners and dental caries (tooth decay)

It has been found that all of the sugars except isomaltulose and tagatose can support the growth of *Streptococcus mutans*, the organism primarily responsible for dental caries. The American Academy of Pediatric Dentistry states that children who have more than three between meal sugar-containing snacks or beverages per day, and children who are put to bed with a bottle containing natural or added sugar are at high risk for dental caries. This applies to both natural and added sugars.

All health claims on food labels are regulated by the FDA in the United States. The FDA has ruled that the sugar alcohols (xylitol, sorbitol, mannitol, maltitol, isomalt, and lactitol) may claim that they do not promote tooth decay. The FDA also allows such a claim for tagatose. Xylitol has been shown in clinical studies to actually inhibit tooth decay, but only at a use level of 5 grams per serving, three times a day [5]. A stick of gum usually has 1 gram or less, so it would take a lot of gum chewing to measurably decrease cavities.

The high potency sweeteners, including acesulfame K, aspartame, saccharin, sucralose, stevia, and the mogrosides of luo han guo, do not support development of dental caries. However, many of the products that contain these sweeteners may contain either acids or sugars that can promote cavity formation.

The Sweeteners

Sweeteners are chemically so diverse that, for years, scientists doubted that they could all work in the same way. We now know that all sweeteners activate the same T1R2/T1R3 taste receptor. I have chosen to sort all sweeteners into four groups.

- Carbohydrates (sugars). This group includes sucrose, glucose, fructose, and lactose. It also includes products like high fructose corn syrup, honey, and agave syrup, that depend on sugars for their sweetness.
- Sugar alcohols (polyols). This group includes sorbitol, erythritol, xylitol, and others. These sweeteners are similar to sugars, but are either undigested or partly digested by humans.
- High potency sweeteners. This group includes acesulfame, aspartame, saccharin, sucralose, and others. These are hundreds or thousands of times as sweet as sucrose, and they do not occur naturally.
- "Natural sweeteners." This group encompasses things that occur in nature, and that are tens or hundreds of times as sweet as sucrose.

This is not a perfect way to sort the sweeteners. Tagatose, for example, is really a sugar, but it is not digested efficiently by humans. Since its adverse effects are more like those of the sugar alcohols, I've put tagatose in that group. Neohesperidin dihydrochalcone is synthesized from a component of citrus fruit, and sucralose is synthesized from sucrose, but both have undergone significant chemical changes, so they do not belong in the "natural sweetener" category. Aspartame is digested to produce three substances that are ubiquitous in the diet, but aspartame itself does not occur in nature, so I have not placed it in the "natural sweeteners" group. And most of the sugars and sugar alcohols are found in nature, but I have separated them from the "natural sweeteners" category.

Carbohydrates (Sugars)

Sugars are the original sweeteners. There are several widely used sugars, including sucrose (table sugar), glucose, fructose, and lactose. In addition, products such as syrups and honey are sweet because of the sugars they contain. Almost all carbohydrates are fully digested, producing 4 calories per gram.

A particular concern for people with diabetes is glucose. People with diabetes need glucose, just as everyone else does, but they must ensure that the blood level stays within safe limits. If a person with diabetes consumes pure glucose, it may be absorbed rapidly, leading to an unsafe blood level. Several of the carbohydrates contain glucose, and some release it rapidly while others do so slowly. Others may be converted to glucose, also at varying rates. The glycemic index provides a measure of the amount of glucose produced and absorbed.

All of the sugars listed in this section can be used in baking. They all can provide bulk, bind water, and participate in the browning reactions that are desirable in baked goods.

Almost all sugars can be utilized by *Streptococcus mutans* (the most common bacteria contributing to tooth decay). Therefore, all of the sugars listed in this section (with the exception of isomaltulose) can contribute to the development of dental caries.

Sucrose

What is it?

Sucrose is ordinary table sugar. It is a *disaccharide*. This means it is made up of two sugar molecules (*monosaccharides*) linked together. Sucrose is formed by linking a glucose and a fructose molecule together. Sucrose is usually refined (purified) from sugar cane or sugar beets. It is also present naturally in many other fruits and plants.

How does it taste?

Sucrose is the standard by which all other sweeteners are judged. It has a clean sweet taste, without bitterness or other off-tastes, and with a fairly fast onset of sweetness. We can detect sweet taste when sucrose is present at a level of 1% or higher. Carbonated soft drinks are commonly sweetened at a level of about 10% sucrose.

How well does it work?

Sucrose is stable in the dry state. When it is used in cooking, it can undergo browning reactions, in which sucrose breaks down to form complex products associated with caramelization. When it is in acidic products (such as many carbonated soft drinks), it may be partly converted to the monosaccharides glucose and fructose. When this happens, it is called inverted sugar. Since both glucose and fructose are sweet, there is no loss of sweetness when this happens.

Sucrose provides other functions in food products in addition to sweetness. It can provide bulk. Depending on the application, it can contribute to crispness, or it can bind moisture to keep foods soft.

How many calories?

Sucrose (and most other sugars) provide 4 calories per gram. It is rapidly digested to glucose and fructose, and these are readily absorbed and metabolized by the body. Sucrose has a glycemic index of 68.

Is it safe?

Sucrose is a naturally occurring carbohydrate that is ubiquitous in the diet. There are enzymes in the body that can readily digest, absorb, and metabolize sucrose, so it is not inherently toxic. It can cause some health problems, however. Consumption of sucrose can promote growth of cavity-forming microorganisms in the mouth, leading to dental caries. For people with diabetes, sucrose can produce excessive blood glucose levels. And *any* carbohydrate (as well as fat or protein), when consumed in excess, can lead to obesity.

Brown sugar, turbinado, molasses

What is it?

When sucrose is extracted from sugar cane or sugar beets, it is refined by repeated evaporation and recrystallization. The juice left behind still contains some sugar. It is called *molasses*. Partially refined sugar, that still has some of this juice stuck to its surface, is called *turbinado sugar* or *raw sugar*. Brown sugar was originally the partially refined sugar, but it is now made by adding controlled amounts of molasses to purified sucrose.

How does it taste?

Brown sugar and turbinado sugar are about as sweet as sucrose, with a characteristic caramel-like flavor from the molasses. Molasses can have some bitterness, and a great deal of flavor in addition to sweetness.

How well does it work?

Brown sugar and turbinado provide about the same amount of sweetness as sucrose. Molasses will be a little less sweet.

How many calories?

Brown sugar has 3.8 calories per gram, slightly lower than sucrose because of the water content of the added molasses. Molasses typically contains about 3 calories per gram. Brown sugar is almost pure sucrose, so it has a glycemic index of 65. Molasses has a glycemic index of 55.

Is it safe?

All of these are metabolized like any other sugar. Molasses may contain some vitamins and minerals that are not present in refined sugar. The amount of vitamins is quite minimal, but there may be significant amounts of calcium, iron, magnesium, or manganese.

Consumption of these sugars can promote growth of cavity-forming microorganisms in the mouth, leading to dental caries. For people with diabetes, they can produce excessive blood glucose levels. Excess calories in any form (carbohydrate, fat, or protein) can lead to obesity.

Fructose

What is it?

Fructose is also known as fruit sugar, because it is present in many fruits. Fructose is one of the building blocks of sucrose, and it is one of the products when sucrose is digested. It is readily metabolized by the human body. Fructose has been used by people with diabetes because it is only slowly converted to glucose, and it does not produce a spike in blood glucose or insulin levels.

How does it taste?

Fructose has a clean sweet taste. It is about 30% sweeter than sucrose, on a weight basis.

How well does it work?

Fructose is the most soluble of the sugars. 4 grams of fructose can dissolve in 1 gram of water. It is far less likely to crystallize than sucrose. It is very hygroscopic (absorbs moisture from the air). It also binds water well in food products, keeping them from drying out too rapidly.

How many calories?

Fructose (and most other sugars) provide 4 calories per gram. It is readily absorbed and metabolized by the body. Fructose has a glycemic index of 15.

Is it safe?

There has been a lot of discussion about the role of fructose (particularly from high fructose corn syrup, HFCS) in obesity. The scientific data show that fructose is neither better nor worse than any other sugar with respect to obesity. As a component of most fruits and honey, fructose has been consumed safely for centuries. There is a safety concern only when too much fructose (or too much of any other caloric substance) is consumed over long periods of time.

Fructose is less cariogenic (cavity-promoting) than sucrose, but it still supports the growth of microorganisms that cause cavities.

Glucose

What is it?

Glucose is also known as dextrose. Glucose is one of the building blocks of sucrose, and it is one of the products when sucrose is digested. Glucose is a major energy source in the human body. It is the *primary* energy source for brain cells. Some glucose can be stored in the body as glycogen, a glucose polymer. Excess glucose can, of course, be converted to fat.

Starches are composed of long chains of glucose molecules linked together. The human digestive system has enzymes that can break starch down into glucose molecules. Food processors can also use enzymes to convert starch into glucose. Corn syrup is an example of this.

How does it taste?

Glucose has a clean sweet taste. It is about 70% as sweet as sucrose, on a weight basis.

How well does it work?

Glucose is less sweet than sucrose, so a larger quantity is needed to provide an equal level of sweetness.

How many calories?

Glucose (and most other sugars) provide 4 calories per gram. It is readily absorbed and metabolized by the body. Glucose has a glycemic index of 100-103.

Is it safe?

Glucose is an important nutrient. It is of particular concern to people with diabetes, who are less able to move excess glucose out of the blood. A high blood glucose level can lead to tissue damage via non-specific glycation (attachment of glucose to proteins in a random manner).

Glucose can support the growth of microorganisms that cause dental caries.

Lactose

What is it?

Lactose is also known as milk sugar, because it is the principal carbohydrate present in milk. It is a disaccharide that is formed by linking a galactose molecule to a glucose molecule.

Human milk contains 6-7% lactose, while cow milk and goat milk contain 4-5% lactose.

How does it taste?

Lactose is about half as sweet as sucrose, on a weight basis, so it is rarely used as a sweetener.

How well does it work?

Lactose is less sweet than sucrose, so a larger quantity would be needed to provide an equal level of sweetness. It is thought that the low level of sweetness provided by lactose in milk encourages the infant to drink the milk.

How many calories?

Lactose (and most other sugars) provides 4 calories per gram. It is readily absorbed and metabolized by infants. Lactose has a glycemic index of 46.

Is it safe?

Infants produce lactase, an enzyme that converts lactose to galactose and glucose. Galactose and glucose are readily absorbed and utilized as energy sources. While some adults continue to produce lactase, others lose the ability to produce this enzyme. When the enzyme is not produced, the human body cannot utilize lactose. The undigested lactose remains in the digestive system, where it is fermented by bacteria, leading to the production of gas and acids that can cause diarrhea. This is the basis of lactose intolerance.

In some yogurts and cheeses, the culture microorganisms utilize some of the lactose for their own growth, decreasing the lactose level in the final product.

Lactose can support the growth of microorganisms that cause dental caries.

Isomaltulose

What is it?

"Isomaltulose" is different from "isomalt," which is covered in the section on sugar alcohols.

Isomaltulose is also known as Palatinose™. It is composed of a glucose molecule and a fructose molecule linked together, much like sucrose. But the linkage is slightly different. The glucose is linked to fructose at carbon atom number six, rather than carbon atom number two (sucrose is glucosyl-1,2-fructose, while isomaltulose is glucosyl-1,6-fructose). Isomaltulose occurs at very low levels in honey and some other food products. It is produced commercially by treating sucrose with an enzyme.

How does it taste?

Isomaltulose is about 40% as sweet as sucrose.

How well does it work?

Isomaltulose can provide some sweetness, and it can participate in browning reactions. It is less sweet than sucrose, so it may be combined with a high potency sweetener. For example, the stevia-based sweetener PureVia™ combines isomaltulose, erythritol, and rebaudioside A.

How many calories?

Isomaltulose provides 4 calories per gram. It is metabolized to glucose and fructose by the body, but the rate of conversion is much slower than for sucrose. The glycemic index of isomaltulose is calculated to be 32.

Is it safe?

Since it is metabolized to glucose and fructose, isomaltulose is as safe as sucrose. Because it is converted more slowly, it does not produce a sharp spike in blood glucose, and it has little or no cariogenic (cavity-promoting) effect on teeth. Isomaltulose has been used in Japan since 1985. It was accepted for use in food by JECFA in 1987, and achieved GRAS status in the United States in 2006.

Corn syrup

What is it?

"Corn syrup" is different from "high fructose corn syrup" (which you can read about in the next section). Corn syrup is produced from corn starch, a polymer of glucose molecules. Depending on the extent to which the starch is broken down, corn syrup may contain varying amounts of glucose, maltose (two glucose molecules linked together), and dextrins (three or more glucoses linked together). Corn syrup contains 15 to 20% glucose.

How does it taste?

Corn syrup has a clean sweet taste. Much of the sweetness comes from glucose, which is 70% as sweet as sucrose. Some sweetness comes from maltose, which is 50% as sweet as sucrose.

How well does it work?

Corn syrup is sweet, but since it is less sweet than sucrose, a larger amount will be needed to provide equivalent sweetness.

How many calories?

Corn syrup provides 4 calories per gram. It is readily absorbed and metabolized by the body. Corn syrup has a glycemic index of 100.

Is it safe?

Corn syrup contains glucose and glucose polymers that can easily be digested to produce glucose. Corn syrup components can support the growth of microorganisms that cause dental caries.

Glucose is an important nutrient, since it is the preferred energy source for the brain. Regulation of the level of glucose in the blood is of concern to people with diabetes. As with any carbohydrate sweetener, excess consumption can lead to obesity.

The glucose in corn syrup can support the growth of microorganisms that cause dental caries.

High fructose corn syrup

What is it?

High fructose corn syrup (HFCS) is made from corn starch. First, the starch (long chains of glucose molecules) is processed with an enzyme that releases the individual glucose molecules. Then it is treated with another enzyme that converts some of the glucose to fructose. The HFCS most commonly used in food products is about 55% fructose and 45% glucose.

How does it taste?

HFCS is commonly used as a replacement for sucrose, and it is quite effective. Fructose is somewhat sweeter than sucrose, and glucose is a little less sweet than sucrose, so the mixture comes quite close to sucrose in sweetness level. The taste quality is also essentially indistinguishable from sucrose.

How well does it work?

HFCS can readily replace sucrose in most food products.

How many calories?

HFCS provides 4 calories per gram. It is readily absorbed and metabolized by the body. HFCS containing 55% fructose is expected to have a glycemic index of 55, based on its fructose and glucose content.

Is it safe?

HFCS is composed of fructose and glucose, both of which are commonly encountered in the diet. There has been a great deal of speculation that HFCS is the cause of the obesity epidemic in the United States. However, obesity is a growing problem in other parts of the world where HFCS is not used. Clinical studies do not show any significant difference between sucrose and HFCS with respect to health. This is not surprising, since both are composed of about equal amounts of glucose and fructose. It is apparent that the problems caused by HFCS are those that are caused by any carbohydrate that is consumed in excess. Excess calories from any source can lead to obesity.

HFCS can support the growth of microorganisms that cause dental caries.

Honey

What is it?

Honey is produced by bees using nectar collected from flowers. It consists mainly of sugars and water, with varying amounts of minerals, amino acids, organic acids, and trace levels of some vitamins. The composition of honey depends on the source of the nectar used by the bees. It is typically about 80% sugars by weight. The main sugars present are fructose and glucose. Some nectars contain sucrose, but the bees digest it to its components, fructose and glucose.

How does it taste?

Honey is very sweet, due to the high level of sugars present. Its taste can be quite variable, depending on the flowers from which it is derived.

How well does it work?

Honey is often used in baking and in other recipes as a replacement for sugar.

How many calories?

Honey has about 3 calories per gram, consistent with its sugar content. The glycemic index depends a great deal on the specific sugars present, and may range from 35 to 87. The average (based on 17 different honeys) is 61.

Is it safe?

Honey has a high enough sugar content to inhibit fermentation and mold growth if it is protected from humidity. Numerous health claims have been made for honey, but most of these have not been investigated under controlled conditions.

Honey can support the growth of microorganisms that cause dental caries.

Agave nectar

What is it?

Agave nectar is produced from the juice of the agave plant. The juice is processed to convert polysaccharides (sugar polymers) into free sugar molecules. The sugar present is mainly fructose, with some glucose. It is then heated to remove some of the water, producing a syrup.

How does it taste?

Agave nectar has a fairly clean sweet taste.

How well does it work?

Since it contains mainly fructose and glucose, agave nectar is a very effective sweetener.

How many calories?

Agave nectar typically has about 3 calories per gram, based on the sugar content. The glycemic index of agave syrup can vary, depending on the source. The average value of the GI is 13.

Is it safe?

Some health benefits have been suggested for agave nectar, primarily because it is "natural." However, it is no more or less healthy than any other sugar. It undergoes processing, just as other sugars do. People with diabetes must account for the carbohydrates present in agave nectar.

Agave syrup can support the growth of microorganisms that cause dental caries.

Sugar alcohols (polyols)

Sugar is important for more than just sweetness in many foods. For example, if you remove the sugar from a cake and replace the sweetness with a high potency sweetener, the cake will be flat and dense and dry. Sugar normally provides bulk and texture, and it holds moisture. Sugar alcohols (also known as polyols) are often referred to as "bulk sweeteners," because they can replace some of the bulk that is missing when sugar is removed from a product.

None of these are in any way related to the alcohol found in beer, wine and spirits. "Alcohol" in this sense is a chemical name for the hydroxyl (-OH) groups that are found in all of the sugars and polyols.

Some polyols occur naturally. Sorbitol, for instance, is found in many fruits. Others are produced by hydrogenating sugars. Xylitol is found in fruits and vegetables, but most of the xylitol used in chewing gum and foods is produced by hydrogenating the sugar xylose, which is extracted from wood or corn cobs.

Polyols provide varying amounts of sweetness. Xylitol is about as sweet as sucrose, maltitol is about 70% as sweet, sorbitol and erythritol are about 60% as sweet, lactitol is about 40% as sweet, and isomalt is about 25% as sweet. Polyols have been used for many years to sweeten products for people with diabetes. While sugars are actively absorbed into the body, polyols are absorbed more slowly. This is important for people with diabetes. They can avoid the rapid rise in blood sugar that would occur with sugar-sweetened foods. Once they are absorbed, many of the polyols can be converted to sugars by the body, so people with diabetes must include sugar alcohols as a source of carbohydrates. The carbohydrates formed from sugar alcohols can produce calories. How many calories? The answer is, "it depends."

First, it depends on how much of the polyol is absorbed. That can vary from person to person, and from day to day. If you eat a very small portion of a polyol, you may be able to absorb almost all of it. If you eat a large quantity, it may not all be absorbed by the time it reaches the large intestine. Once it reaches the large intestine, it's fair game for the bacteria that live there. If they consume the calories, you don't! But if they consume it, other things happen, as described below.

Second, the calorie content depends on how efficiently your body can convert the polyol to sugars. Sorbitol and xylitol are converted to sugars quite efficiently, while mannitol is not.

So the calories listed on the label are based on results of scientific studies, mainly in experimental animals. At best, they are a rough estimate of the number of calories you can expect to get from the product. The table below lists the values currently accepted by the FDA for commonly used polyols (in the European Union, most polyols are listed at 2.4 calories per gram).

Polyol	Calories per gram
Sorbitol	2.6
Xylitol	2.4
Maltitol	2.1
Isomalt	2.0
Lactitol	2.0
Mannitol	1.6
Erythritol	0.2

Now the bad news. Polyols provide fewer calories per gram than carbohydrates because they are not efficiently absorbed and metabolized by humans. When polyols are consumed in large quantity, the unabsorbed and unmetabolized materials can have a variety of effects when they reach the large intestine. Symptoms may range from borborygmus (an interesting word that describes gastric rumbling sounds!) to gas, abdominal pain, and diarrhea.

Many of the polyols can have an *osmotic* effect, as they attract and bind water. When a large quantity of polyol attracts a lot of water into the large intestine, the result may be diarrhea. Laxatives such as polyethylene glycol (MiraLAX®) and magnesium sulfate (milk of magnesia) work in just this way.

In addition, the undigested polyols may be metabolized by the microorganisms that inhabit the large intestine. When this happens, one of the products may be gas, so flatulence is a common result. Microbial metabolism can also produce short chain fatty acids. These can also have osmotic effects.

There is a lot of individual variation. Some people suffer a lot, and some not at all. Some people do well with one polyol and not with another. It depends on the quantity consumed, it depends on your body and your personal collection of intestinal bacteria, and it depends on how often you use the products. People can develop a tolerance to the polyols, as their bodies and their bacterial populations adapt.

There have been clinical studies performed to determine the "laxative threshold values" (LTV) for many of the polyols. The LTV is the amount that may cause a laxative effect if consumed in a single meal by a normal, unadapted adult. The table below lists some representative results. There is some variation in the values, because different studies use different ways to measure the effect.

Polyol	Laxative Threshold Value
Maltitol	60 g
Erythritol	40
Isomalt	29
Lactitol	24–50
Sorbitol	23
Xylitol	20
Mannitol	10–20

Adapted from Levin et al., Sugar substitutes: their energy values, bulk characteristics, and potential health benefits. Am. J. Clin. Nutr. 62(suppl):1161S-1168S (1995).

When you consume polyols, read labels carefully, and pay attention to quantities consumed. Your results may vary, for the reasons discussed above!

The polyols in this section can substitute for sugars in many baking applications. They provide bulk, and they bind water. However, they cannot participate in the browning reactions that give baked goods their characteristic color, and they cannot undergo caramelization as sugars do.

Sorbitol

What is it?

Sorbitol is also known as glucitol. It is found in many fruits, including apples, pears, cherries, and plums. It has the European Registry Number E420.

How does it taste?

Sorbitol has a clean sweet taste. It is about 60% as sweet as sucrose.

How well does it work?

Sorbitol behaves much like sucrose in food systems, with respect to providing bulk and interacting with other components to produce suitable texture. It is particularly good at binding moisture (humectant activity).

Sorbitol and the other polyols generally do not participate in browning reactions that provide characteristic color to baked goods.

How many calories?

Sorbitol is slowly absorbed by humans. It can be converted to glucose in the body, but this is a slow process, so it does not produce a glucose spike in people with diabetes. In the United States, sorbitol provides 2.6 calories per gram for labeling purposes. In the European Union, it is listed at 2.4 calories per gram. Sorbitol has a glycemic index of 9.

Is it safe?

Unabsorbed sorbitol can cause some negative side effects in the digestive system, including gas, rumbling sounds (borborygmus), and diarrhea, depending on the amount used and individual sensitivity. The Joint FAO/WHO Expert Committee on Food Additives (JECFA) has determined the "Laxative Threshold Value" (LTV) for a number of polyols, and sorbitol is one of the more laxative polyols with an LTV of 23 grams per meal. The FDA requires the following label statement for foods whose reasonably foreseeable consumption may result in the daily ingestion of 50 grams of sorbitol: "Excess consumption may have a laxative effect."

Sorbitol does not support the growth of microorganisms that cause dental caries.

Isomalt

What is it?

"Isomalt" is different from "isomaltulose," which is covered in the section on sugars.

Isomalt is produced from sucrose in two steps: enzymatic rearrangement of sucrose to isomaltulose, followed by hydrogenation. It is a mixture of two compounds, glucosyl-mannitol and glucosyl-sorbitol. Isomalt is sold under the trade name Palatinit™. It has the European Registry Number E953.

How does it taste?

Isomalt has a clean sweet taste. It is about 40% as sweet as sucrose, on a weight basis.

How well does it work?

Isomalt's physical properties are very similar to sucrose, making it useful in hard candies and many other products. It is less hygroscopic (less likely to pick up moisture from the air) than most polyols and sugars, so products made with isomalt may be less sticky and may have a better shelf life. Isomalt has very good heat stability, so it can be used in making hard candies and baked goods.

How many calories?

Isomalt is not efficiently absorbed by the body, and it is only partly metabolized. Its caloric value depends on several factors. In the United States, isomalt provides 2 calories per gram for labeling purposes. In the European Union, it is listed at 2.4 calories per gram. Isomalt has a glycemic index of 9.

Is it safe?

Isomalt has GRAS status in the United States. It has been in use in Europe for over 20 years.

The Joint FAO/WHO Expert Committee on Food Additives has determined the "Laxative Threshold Value" (LTV) for a number of polyols, and isomalt has an LTV of 29 grams per meal.

Isomalt does not support the growth of microorganisms that cause dental caries.

Lactitol

What is it?

Lactitol is produced by hydrogenation of lactose. It is also known as galactosyl-glucitol. It has the European Registry Number E966.

How does it taste?

Lactitol is about 40% as sweet as sucrose. It produces a menthol-like cooling effect in the mouth.

How well does it work?

Lactitol is not hygroscopic (does not absorb moisture from the air), so it is useful in products where crispness is desirable. It also performs well in chocolate. It has very good stability and solubility.

How many calories?

Lactitol is not efficiently absorbed by the body, and it is only partly metabolized. Its caloric value depends on several factors. In the United States, lactitol provides 2 calories per gram for labeling purposes. In the European Union, it is listed at 2.4 calories per gram. Lactitol has a glycemic index of 4.

Is it safe?

Lactitol has GRAS status in the United States. It is approved for use in the European Union, Canada, Japan, and several other countries.

The Joint FAO/WHO Expert Committee on Food Additives has determined the "Laxative Threshold Value" (LTV) for a number of polyols, and lactitol has an LTV of 24-50 grams per meal.

Lactitol does not support the growth of microorganisms that cause dental caries.

Maltitol

What is it?

Maltitol is produced by hydrogenation of the disaccharide maltose. It has the European Registry Number E965.

How does it taste?

Maltitol is about 70% as sweet as sucrose. It also produces a very slight cooling feeling in the mouth.

How well does it work?

Maltitol is not very hygroscopic, so it performs well in chocolate and other low-moisture foods. Like the other polyols, maltitol does not participate in browning reactions.

How many calories?

Maltitol is only partially absorbed by the body, and it is only partly metabolized. Its caloric value depends on several factors. In the United States, maltitol provides 2.1 calories per gram for labeling purposes. In the European Union, it is listed at 2.4 calories per gram. Maltitol has a glycemic index of 35.

Is it safe?

Maltitol has GRAS status in the United States. It is approved for use in the European Union.

The Joint FAO/WHO Expert Committee on Food Additives has determined the "Laxative Threshold Value" (LTV) for a number of polyols, and maltitol is one of the less laxative polyols with an LTV of 60 grams per meal.

Maltitol does not support the growth of microorganisms that cause dental caries.

Mannitol

What is it?

Mannitol is found in mushrooms, algae, seaweeds, and trees. It can also be produced by hydrogenation of fructose. It has the European Registry Number E421.

How does it taste?

Mannitol is about 50% as sweet as sucrose. It produces a menthol-like cooling effect in the mouth.

How well does it work?

Unlike sorbitol, mannitol does not bind water well. It is used as a dusting powder on chewing gums. It has a high heat stability and can be used in chocolate flavored coatings.

How many calories?

Mannitol is not efficiently absorbed by the body, and it is only partly metabolized. Its caloric value depends on several factors. In the United States, mannitol provides 1.6 calories per gram for labeling purposes. In the European Union, it is listed at 2.4 calories per gram. Mannitol has a glycemic index of 0.

Is it safe?

Mannitol occurs naturally in many plants. The FDA permits use of mannitol in the United States. The Joint Food and Agriculture Organization/World Health Organization Expert Committee on Food Additives (JECFA) has concluded that mannitol is safe.

The Joint FAO/WHO Expert Committee on Food Additives has determined the "Laxative Threshold Value" (LTV) for a number of polyols. It estimates the LTV for mannitol to be between 10 and 20 grams per meal. The FDA requires the following label statement for foods whose reasonably foreseeable consumption may result in the daily ingestion of 20 grams of mannitol: "Excess consumption may have a laxative effect."

Mannitol does not support the growth of microorganisms that cause dental caries.

Xylitol

What is it?

Xylitol occurs naturally in fruits and vegetables, but most of the xylitol used in chewing gum and foods is produced by hydrogenating the sugar xylose, which is extracted from wood or corn cobs. It has the European Registry Number E967.

How does it taste?

Xylitol is about equal in sweetness to sucrose. It also produces a cooling feeling in the mouth.

How well does it work?

Xylitol is used primarily in chewing gums and confections, where the cooling effect is not a serious drawback.

How many calories?

Xylitol is not efficiently absorbed by the body, and it is only partly metabolized. Its caloric value depends on several factors. In the United States, xylitol provides 2.4 calories per gram for labeling purposes. In the European Union, it is also listed at 2.4 calories per gram. Xylitol has a glycemic index of 13.

Is it safe?

The Joint FAO/WHO Expert Committee on Food Additives has determined the "Laxative Threshold Value" (LTV) for a number of polyols, and xylitol has an LTV of 20 grams per meal.

Xylitol is used extensively in chewing gum. In general, polyols are permitted by the FDA to claim that they do not promote dental caries, but xylitol has been shown to *reduce* the incidence of dental caries. However, you would need to use 5 to 6 grams of xylitol, 3 times a day, to have a clinical effect [5], and a stick of gum typically contains 1 gram or less. Xylitol is not efficiently used by bacteria, so it slows their growth and inhibits acid production. It also appears to prevent adhesion, by decreasing production of insoluble biofilm. Finally, when used in chewing gum, xylitol stimulates saliva flow, and increased saliva flow also inhibits carie formation.

Xylitol is particularly toxic for dogs. It is readily absorbed by dogs, and it rapidly raises insulin levels and causes liver damage. So keep xylitol-sweetened gum and candy out of reach of your pets!

Inulin and Fructooligosaccharides

What is it?

Inulins are carbohydrate polymers composed mainly of fructose molecules linked together in chains, with small amounts of glucose as well. Fructooligosaccharides are shorter chains of fructose molecules, usually with one glucose molecule attached. Fructooligosaccharides are prepared by enzymatically attaching one or more fructose molecules to a sucrose molecule, or by partially breaking down inulin with enzymes.

Inulin and fructooligosaccharides are described as "prebiotics," meaning that they support the growth of bacteria that are considered beneficial in the digestive system. Note the possible effects of prebiotics in the "Is it safe?" section below. Inulin is added to foods as a source of fiber.

How does it taste?

Inulin has a low level of sweetness, perhaps 10% as sweet as sucrose on a weight basis. Fructooligosaccharides are about 30% as sweet as sucrose.

How well does it work?

Inulin and fructooligosaccharides can replace some of the physical characteristics of sucrose, such as binding water and providing bulk. They are not sweet enough on their own to replace sucrose as a sweetener in most situations.

How many calories?

Inulin and fructooligosaccharides are only partially digested, so they provide less calories than other carbohydrates. Inulin is reported to provide 1–1.5 calories per gram. Studies of fructooligosaccharides have provided values of 1.0–2.8 calories per gram. Current nutrition labels use values of 1.5–1.7 calories per gram.

Is it safe?

Inulin is a natural component of many plants, including garlic, onion, chicory, and agave. It has GRAS status in the United States. Since it is a complex carbohydrate and it is only partly digested by human digestive enzymes, it is a good substrate for microorganisms that live in the digestive system. These organisms may ferment the inulin, producing gas and, in some cases, diarrhea.

Some fructooligosaccharides also occur naturally, while others do not. Fructooligosaccharides have been used in Japan since 1989, and they have GRAS status in the United States. Fructooligosaccharides are also only partly digested and can support the growth of microorganisms, so they can also produce gas and diarrhea if consumed in excess.

It is not clear whether inulin and fructooligosaccharides promote dental caries.

Tagatose

What is it?

Tagatose is a monosaccharide that is chemically similar to fructose. It occurs naturally (at low levels) in some yogurts, as it is a metabolic intermediate of lactobacilli. It has GRAS status in the United States. The Joint FAO/WHO Expert Committee on Food Additives (JECFA) has approved tagatose as a "novel food ingredient", with no limitation on its usage.

How does it taste?

Tagatose has a clean sweet taste. It is about 90% as sweet as sucrose, on a weight basis.

How well does it work?

Tagatose can function well as a sweetener. In addition to sweetness, it provides bulk and water-binding characteristics, and it can undergo browning reactions which are important in baking applications.

How many calories?

Tagatose is only partly absorbed by the body, and not converted to energy very efficiently. Its caloric value depends on several factors. In the United States, tagatose provides 1.5 calories per gram for labeling purposes. In the European Union, it is listed at 2.4 calories per gram. Tagatose has a glycemic index of 3.

Is it safe?

Since it is not efficiently absorbed and digested, tagatose may remain in the digestive system, where it can be fermented by bacteria. This can lead to production of gas and acids, which may produce diarrhea if tagatose is consumed in large quantities.

Tagatose does not support the growth of cavity-causing bacteria in the mouth. In the United States, the FDA allows tagatose to claim that it does not promote tooth decay (but it cannot claim to be sugar free because it is actually a sugar).

Erythritol

What is it?

Erythritol is a polyol that occurs naturally at low levels in some fruits, mushrooms, and fermented foods such as wine, soy sauce, and cheese. It has the European Registry Number E968.

How does it taste?

Erythritol is about 70% as sweet as sucrose, on a weight basis. It produces a cooling effect in the mouth, similar to xylitol.

How well does it work?

Erythritol is not hygroscopic (does not pick up moisture from the air). It has lower water solubility than sucrose and a higher tendency to crystallize.

How many calories?

Unlike other polyols, erythritol is readily absorbed in the small intestine. It is not readily metabolized in the human body, so it provides only 0.2 calories per gram. Erythritol has a glycemic index of 0.

Is it safe?

Erythritol has been used in Japan since 1990 and has had GRAS status in the United States since 1996. It received approval for some uses from the European Union in 2008.

Erythritol is largely absorbed in the small intestine and excreted in the urine. It is not metabolized in the body. Since most of it is absorbed, it is not subject to fermentation in the large intestine as most polyols are. This means there is far less gas-forming and laxative effect, compared to the other polyols. One study reported that a 50 g dose produced some rumbling (borborygmus), but no diarrhea [6].

Erythritol does not support the development of dental caries. Some research suggests that it may, under some conditions, actually inhibit the growth of oral bacteria that cause tooth decay, but this has not been shown with certainty.

Glycerol

What is it?

Glycerol (also known as glycerin or glycerine) is a component of triglycerides (fats). It can be used by the body to make fats, or it can be metabolized as a carbohydrate. It has the European Registry Number E422.

How does it taste?

Glycerol is about 60% as sweet as sucrose, on a weight basis.

How well does it work?

Glycerol is less sweet than sucrose, and it provides as many calories per gram as sucrose, so it has little use as a sweetener. It is more often used for its ability to bind moisture and to keep food products moist.

How many calories?

Unlike most other polyols, glycerol is readily absorbed in the small intestine. It is also easily metabolized, producing about 4 calories per gram. Glycerol has a glycemic index of 0.

Is it safe?

Glycerol is widely used as an ingredient in processed foods. It is a natural component of all living cells, so it has very low toxicity. In a study involving 8 healthy human subjects, a 35 gram sample of glycerol was well tolerated, while a 75 gram sample caused mild nausea or headache for 4 of the subjects.

It is not clear whether glycerol has any effect, positive or negative, on dental caries.

High Potency Sweeteners

In this section, we look at compounds that are much sweeter than sucrose, on a weight basis. The naturally occurring high potency sweeteners, such as stevioside, are in a separate section, for convenience.

Some of these sweeteners are so much more potent than sucrose, that it is difficult to measure them out in single serving quantities. For example, a packet of Splenda™ contains about 1% sucralose and 99% maltodextrin (starch, a polymer of glucose). Without the maltodextrin, it would be very hard to put the correct amount of sucralose into each packet, and it would also be hard to get all of the sucralose out when you want to use it. Of course the maltodextrin has 4 calories per gram, but the amount present is only about a gram. If the packet has less than 5 calories, the FDA allows for a zero calorie claim.

Glycemic index is not measured for most high potency sweeteners, because it is understood that (a) glycemic index is based on carbohydrate content, and most high potency sweeteners do not contain carbohydrate, and (b) most high potency sweeteners cannot produce glucose, and (c) their use level is so low that any glucose produced would be negligible. I list a GI value of 0 for these sweeteners, but these values are not based on actual experimentation. It would be unpleasant and impractical to ask a human being to consume 25 or 50 grams of any of these substances, and the resulting number would be meaningless.

Most high potency sweeteners have one or more off tastes. There is a real advantage in combining two or more different sweeteners, because the sweetness is additive, and the different off tastes are not. This is why Pepsi Next™ uses a combination of four different sweeteners. It is possible to achieve 60% calorie reduction while minimizing off tastes due to sweeteners.

The sweeteners in this section can provide sweetness in many baking applications, but they cannot provide the bulk or browning reactions that sugars do. In commercial products, these sweeteners are often combined with sugar alcohols, because the sugar alcohols can provide the bulk and bind moisture. The exception in this group is aspartame, which can lose its sweetness when heated. Aspartame can be used to sweeten a cup of coffee, but not the prolonged heating in a baking process.

Acesulfame potassium

What is it?

Acesulfame potassium (also known as acesulfame, acesulfame K or Ace-K) is the potassium salt of 6-Methyl-3,4-dihydro-1,2,3-oxathiazin-4-one 2,2-dioxide. It is sold under the trade names Sunett™ and Sweet One™. It has the European Registry Number E950.

How does it taste?

Acesulfame has a sweet taste. Many people experience a bitter-metallic aftertaste (much like saccharin). Its onset of sweetness is rapid. The sweetness potency relative to sucrose is about 200, but depends upon the concentration of sucrose which is being matched.

How well does it work?

Acesulfame potassium has high water solubility. Some people experience a clean sweet taste, while others notice a strong bitter metallic off-taste. This is due to differences in certain bitter taste receptors. Because of the high incidence of bitter taste, acesulfame is rarely used as the sole sweetener in foods and beverages. It is usually blended with one or more other sweeteners to minimize off-tastes. Acesulfame potassium has good stability in foods and beverages.

How many calories?

Acesulfame has no caloric content. Its glycemic index is 0.

Is it safe?

Acesulfame is a small molecule with high water solubility. It is rapidly absorbed by the body and then rapidly excreted in the urine. Acesulfame has been approved by the FDA, the EFSA in Europe, and JECFA. The FDA and JECFA have established an ADI of 15 milligrams per kilogram of body weight per day, and EFSA has set the ADI at 9 milligrams per kilogram of body weight per day.

Acesulfame does not support the growth of microorganisms that cause dental caries.

Aspartame

What is it?

Aspartame is L-aspartyl-L-phenylalanine methyl ester. It is composed of two amino acids (aspartate and phenylalanine) and a methyl ester. Amino acids are the building blocks from which all proteins are made. Aspartame is sold under the trade names NutraSweet™, Equal™, and Canderel™. It has the European Registry Number E951.

How does it taste?

Aspartame has a clean sweet taste, with little or no bitterness for most people. Its onset of sweetness may be very slightly slower than sucrose, and the sweetness may linger somewhat longer than sucrose.

How well does it work?

The stability of aspartame in the dry state is very good. In food systems, the main limitation of aspartame is its tendency to lose sweetness at high temperature. When water is present, it can undergo hydrolysis (the same thing that happens when it is digested, as described below). This makes it tasteless, and unsuitable for most baking applications. The rate of breakdown with heat is not so rapid as to prevent its use in sweetening coffee, tea, or other hot drinks. The rate of breakdown also depends on pH (acidity). Most baked goods are near neutral pH, where aspartame stability is not as good. Aspartame is most stable at pH 4-5, a level of acidity that is found in many soft drinks.

How many calories?

Since it is made up of amino acids, aspartame has about 4 calories per gram, just like protein. But it has about 180 times the sweetness potency of sucrose, so the amount used in foods and beverages is very small. Therefore, it adds only 1 or 2 calories to the diet in most foods and beverages. For example, a 12 ounce diet soft drink might contain about 125 mg (0.125 gram) of aspartame, which would have less than 1 calorie. In contrast, a 12 ounce sugar-sweetened soft drink would have about 25 grams of sugar and about 100 calories. Its glycemic index is 0.

Is it safe?

Aspartame has been approved by the FDA in the United States, the EFSA in Europe, and JECFA. The FDA has established an ADI of 50 milligrams per kilogram of body weight per day. EFSA and JECFA have set the ADI at 40 milligrams per kilogram of body weight per day.

Aspartame does not support the growth of microorganisms that cause dental caries.

When aspartame is consumed, it is converted by digestive enzymes to three components: aspartate, phenylalanine, and methanol (methyl alcohol).

Aspartate is an amino acid that is present in every protein we consume, and in every protein in the human body. It is also an intermediate in metabolizing carbohydrates and other amino acids. The human body can make it from other substances if it needs to, and it can burn it for energy or convert it to fat if there is more than enough.

Phenylalanine is another amino acid that is present in all proteins. In contrast to aspartic acid, humans cannot produce it from other materials. We must get a certain amount of it every day in our diet, so it is classified as an essential amino acid. If we consume more than we need, we can burn the excess for energy, or store the extra calories as fat. Phenylalanine is only a concern for people with the rare genetic disorder phenylketonuria (PKU). PKU is a condition that is detected at birth with a screening test. People with PKU lack the enzyme to break down excess phenylalanine, so they must carefully monitor their phenylalanine intake. They still need a certain amount of it to make proteins, but they must be careful not to consume more than this amount. For this reason, products containing aspartame display a warning label for people with phenylketonuria.

What about the *methanol*? Isn't methanol poisonous? Methanol is present in a lot of fruits and fruit juices, partly in the form of methyl esters, including pectin. In the digestive system, many of these esters are hydrolyzed to release methanol. Your liver is equipped to handle methanol in this kind of quantity. It oxidizes the methanol to formaldehyde and then to formic acid, which is easily handled by the kidneys. The enzymes doing this are alcohol dehydrogenase and aldehyde dehydrogenase. The process is so efficient that you would have a hard time measuring any formaldehyde in your body. This is true whether you get the methanol from a glass of tomato juice (85 mg), apple juice (21 mg), or a can of diet cola (20 mg).

Remember what the toxicologists say: "the dose makes the poison." Methanol becomes toxic when you start consuming large quantities, e.g., if you drink enough of it to become intoxicated. Now you overwhelm the amount of oxidative enzymes present in the liver, measurable quantities of formaldehyde accumulate, and you generate enough formic acid to upset the acid-base balance of the body. But here we are talking about tens of grams of methanol, about a thousand times more than you could get by consuming tomatoes, apples or diet cola.

One of the internet myths is that fruit juices are different because they contain small amounts of ethanol, and the ethanol is an antidote to methanol poisoning. It is true that, in the case of a patient who has acute methanol poisoning, one of the treatments is to administer ethanol. The rationale is that the ethanol will compete with methanol for the attention of those oxidative enzymes, and you will get less formic acid (methanol oxidation product) and more acetic acid (ethanol oxidation product). The human body can convert acetic acid to fat. You would not get enough ethanol in fruits and vegetables to have this kind of effect, so calling the ethanol in fruit juice an "antidote" is a gross misrepresentation.

Neohesperidin dihydrochalcone

What is it?

Neohesperidin dihydrochalcone is also known as neo-DHC. It is synthesized by chemical treatment of neohesperidin, a bitter component of bitter orange, grapefruit, and other citrus fruit peel and pulp. It has the European Registry Number E959 and FEMA GRAS number 3811.

How does it taste?

Neohesperidin dihydrochalcone is up to 1000 times as sweet as sucrose, but it has a number of other properties that limit its use as a sweetener. First, it has an intense cooling effect on the tongue. Second, it has licorice-like and bitter off-tastes. Third, it is slow in onset and has a lingering taste that make it decidedly not sucrose-like.

How well does it work?

Neohesperidin dihydrochalcone has poor water solubility, but good stability in foods and beverages. It has several off-tastes, so it is often used in combination with one or more other sweeteners to minimize the off-tastes. It can mask some bitter tastes. It is also used in some situations as a flavor enhancer.

How many calories?

Neohesperidin dihydrochalcone has no caloric value. Its glycemic index is 0.

Is it safe?

Neohesperidin dihydrochalcone is approved for use in Europe, but is not formally approved in the United States. The Flavor and Extract Manufacturers Association (FEMA) has self-affirmed neohesperidin dihydrochalcone as GRAS in the United States. EFSA has established an ADI of 5 milligrams per kilogram of body weight per day. JECFA has not evaluated neohesperidin dihydrochalcone.

Neohesperidin dihydrochalcone does not support the growth of microorganisms that cause dental caries.

Neotame

What is it?

Neotame is also known as neohexyl aspartame. It consists of an aspartame molecule to which a six carbon chain has been added. It has the European Registry Number E961.

How does it taste?

Neotame is sweet, with a potency about 8,000 times sucrose, on a weight basis. There is little or no off-taste, except that, at high sweetness levels, it has a slight licorice-like cooling effect in the mouth. Its sweetness is slower in onset than sucrose, and it lingers significantly at high sweetness levels.

How well does it work?

Neotame is a highly potent sweetener, so use levels are very low. It has better stability than aspartame. Like aspartame, its stability is pH-dependent, with optimum stability at about pH 4.5. Its stability is also temperature dependent, but it is sufficiently heat stable to work in baking applications. Its water solubility is 12.6 grams/liter at 25°C. Because of its slow onset, neotame is usually blended with another sweetener (such as aspartame, acesulfame, or saccharin) that has a fast onset.

How many calories?

Neotame has no caloric value. Its glycemic index is 0.

Is it safe?

Neotame was approved by the FDA in 2002 for use in the United States. JECFA confirmed the safety of neotame in 2003. It is approved in Australia and New Zealand, and a number of countries in Europe and South America. The FDA established an ADI of 18 milligrams per day. JECFA and EFSA have set an ADI of 2 milligrams per kilogram of body weight per day.

Neotame has no effect on blood glucose or insulin levels.

Neotame produces insignificant amounts of methanol and phenylalanine when metabolized. Consumption of neotame is not a concern for people with the rare genetic condition, *phenylketonuria*, who must monitor their intake of the essential amino acid, phenylalanine.

Neotame does not support the growth of microorganisms that cause dental caries.

Saccharin

What is it?

Saccharin is an organic acid. It is most commonly used as the sodium salt. The calcium salt and free saccharin are also used. In the United States, Sweet'N Low™ and Sugar Twin™ contain sodium saccharin. Saccharin has the European Registry Number E954.

How does it taste?

Saccharin has a sweet taste. Many (but not all) people experience a bitter-metallic off taste. Its onset of sweetness is rapid. The sweetness potency relative to sucrose is about 300, but it depends upon the concentration of sucrose which is being matched.

How well does it work?

Saccharin (as the sodium or calcium salt) is quite water soluble. Because of its significant bitterness for many consumers, it is often used in combination with other sweeteners, to minimize off-tastes.

How many calories?

Saccharin has no caloric value. Its glycemic index is 0.

Is it safe?

Saccharin is very water-soluble. It is slowly absorbed from the intestine, and rapidly excreted in the urine.

Saccharin does not support the growth of microorganisms that cause dental caries.

Saccharin is approved for use by the FDA, JECFA, and EFSA. All three agencies have established an ADI of 5 milligrams per kilogram of body weight per day.

Saccharin was discovered in 1879 and was in use as a sweetener in the United States in 1906 when the first Pure Food and Drug Act was passed by Congress. Harvey Wiley, the first Commissioner of the Food and Drug Administration, wanted to ban saccharin because it deceived consumers into thinking they were getting sugar, when they were not (this was before detailed ingredient labels were required). President Theodore Roosevelt, a daily user of saccharin, overruled Wiley, stating, "Anybody who says saccharin is injurious to health is an idiot."

Saccharin was widely used in the United States during World War I because of sugar shortages, and the rise of diet foods and beverages in the 1960s further increased usage. During this period, it was considered to be "generally recognized as safe" (GRAS).

In the late 1960s, studies of cyclamate and saccharin in rats suggested links to bladder tumors. This led to a ban of cyclamate in the United States, and a ban of saccharin in Canada. The Delaney Clause of the Food and Drug Act, enacted in 1958, mandated the banning of any substance that could induce cancer in animals, so the FDA moved to ban saccharin. However, the lack of alternative low calorie sweeteners at the time led to public opposition to this action. Congress responded by allowing saccharin to remain on the market, but requiring products containing saccharin to carry the warning "USE OF THIS PRODUCT MAY BE HAZARDOUS TO YOUR HEALTH. THIS PRODUCT CONTAINS SACCHARIN WHICH HAS BEEN DETERMINED TO CAUSE CANCER IN LABORATORY ANIMALS."

In 1996, it was reported by the American Health Foundation that a combination of sodium saccharin with high pH, high calcium phosphate concentration, and high protein concentration (which is unique to male rats) causes formation of a solid material in the rat bladder [7]. This material damages the rat's bladder and provokes overactive regrowth of bladder cells. This phenomenon has not been observed in mice or in any other species, including humans. Thus, it is likely that saccharin is carcinogenic only in male rats, and that it is quite safe for humans. In 2000, the warning label requirement was lifted.

Sucralose

What is it?

Sucralose is also known as 1',4,6'-trichloro-galactosucrose. It is a sucrose molecule in which three of the -OH groups have been replaced by chlorine atoms. In the course of the chlorination, the stereochemistry at position 4 of the glucose ring gets inverted, so it is named as a derivative of *galacto-* sucrose. Sucralose has the European Registry Number E955.

How does it taste?

Sucralose tastes sweet, with a slight off-taste that is described as "drying" or bitter by some tasters. It has a slightly slower onset of sweetness than sucrose, and the sweetness lingers a little longer than sucrose. The sweetness potency relative to sucrose is about 600, but it depends upon the concentration of sucrose which is being matched.

How well does it work?

Sucralose is relatively stable, and can be used in baking.

How many calories?

Sucralose has no caloric value. Its glycemic index is 0.

Is it safe?

Sucralose was approved by the Food and Drug Administration in 1998, and by the European Union in 2004. The FDA has set an ADI of 5 milligrams per kilogram of body weight per day. JECFA and EFSA have set an ADI of 15 milligrams per kilogram of body weight per day. Sucralose is only partially absorbed, and the absorbed sucralose is excreted by the kidneys.

Sucralose does not support the growth of microorganisms that cause dental caries.

Cyclamate

What is it?
Cyclamate is usually sold as the sodium or calcium salt of cyclamic acid (also known as cyclohexylsulfamic acid). In Canada, Sugar Twin™ and Equal™ Cyclamate contain sodium cyclamate. Cyclamate has the European Registry Number E952.

How does it taste?
Cyclamate is 30 to 50 times as sweet as sucrose. It has a sweet taste. Some people can detect a low level of bitterness. At high use levels, it may taste slightly salty as well.

How well does it work?
Cyclamate has good water solubility, and good stability in foods and beverages. It has relatively low potency compared to other sweeteners, and is often used in combination with one or more other sweeteners to minimize off-tastes.

How many calories?
Cyclamate has no caloric value. Its glycemic index is 0.

Is it safe?
In 1958, cyclamate was granted GRAS status in the United States. However, a 1968 study suggested a link to bladder tumors in rats. This led to a ban of cyclamate in the United States. It has been found that saccharin causes bladder tumors in rats by the formation of a solid material in the rat bladder at high doses (see Saccharin, on page 54). Since cyclamate and saccharin are both negatively charged organic molecules that are rapidly excreted in the urine, it may be that cyclamate provokes a response in rats similar to saccharin.

Cyclamate is currently approved in Europe, Australia, Canada, Mexico, and much of South America. However, it is not approved for use in the United States. It is largely excreted unchanged in the urine, although varying amounts (usually 0-3%) may be converted to cyclohexylamine before excretion. Cyclohexylamine is known to be toxic at some levels, but it is not likely that the amount produced from dietary intake would cause toxicity to humans. JECFA has set an ADI of 11 milligrams per kilogram of body weight per day. EFSA has set an ADI of 7 milligrams per kilogram of body weight per day.

Cyclamate does not support the growth of microorganisms that cause dental caries.

Alitame

What is it?

Alitame is chemically related to aspartame. It retains the aspartic acid component, but the phenylalanine methyl ester is replaced by a non-natural D-alanine amide. Alitame has the European Registry Number E956. It was sold in some countries until 2008, when the manufacturer discontinued production because of high material costs.

How does it taste?

Alitame tastes sweet. The sweetness potency relative to sucrose is about 2000, but it depends upon the concentration of sucrose which is being matched.

How well does it work?

Alitame has better heat stability than aspartame.

How many calories?

Alitame could, in principle, release aspartic acid, which has caloric value. Due to the high sweetness potency of alitame, the amount of aspartic acid would be minimal, contributing one calorie or less in typical food or beverage applications. Its glycemic index is 0.

Is it safe?

Alitame is not approved for use in the United States. It has been approved for use in Mexico, Australia, New Zealand, and China. JECFA established an ADI of 1 milligram per kilogram of body weight per day.

Alitame does not support the growth of microorganisms that cause dental caries.

Other Natural Products

This group consists of several naturally occurring materials that are tens or hundreds of times as sweet as sucrose. Please keep in mind that "natural" is not a synonym for "safe"! Cholera toxin occurs in nature, and it is deadly. Many of these substances have been used for hundreds of years, but that also does not guarantee 100% safety. See, for example, glycyrrhizin, the sweet component of licorice root, which can be anti-inflammatory, but can also cause serious water retention that would be dangerous for a person with high blood pressure.

As with the other high potency sweeteners, glycemic index (GI) is not measured for these sweeteners, because it is understood that (a) glycemic index is based on carbohydrate content, and most high potency sweeteners do not contain carbohydrate, and (b) most high potency sweeteners cannot produce glucose, and (c) their use level is so low that any glucose produced would be negligible. I list a GI value of 0 for these sweeteners, but these values are not based on actual experimentation. It would be unpleasant and impractical to ask a human being to consume 25 or 50 grams of any of these substances, and the resulting number would be meaningless.

The sweeteners in this section can provide sweetness in many baking applications, but they cannot provide the bulk or browning reactions that sugars do. In commercial products, these sweeteners are sometimes combined with sugar alcohols, because the sugar alcohols can provide the bulk and bind moisture. The exceptions in this group are monellin and curculin, which may lose their sweetness when heated.

Some of the sweeteners in this section are not yet commercially available, but are being developed for consumer use.

Stevia, stevioside, and rebaudioside

What is it?

Stevia (*Stevia rebaudiana* Bertoni) is a plant native to Paraguay and Brazil. It goes by a number of names, including sweet leaf, sweet herb, sweet herb of Paraguay, candyleaf, honey leaf, sweet honey leaf, and honey yerba. The leaves are used by the native Guaraní people to sweeten food and drinks. The plant is grown commercially in Paraguay, Brazil, and China. It produces at least six different sweet-tasting compounds: stevioside, rebaudioside A, rebaudioside C, rebaudioside D, rebaudioside E, and dulcoside A. These compounds are diterpene glycosides. They are sometimes referred to as *steviol glycosides*, because they are composed of the diterpene *steviol* with various sugars attached.

Stevia can be used in the form of fresh or dried leaves, or the sweet terpenes can be extracted. The extracts can be further purified to produce either a mixture of the sweet terpenes, or to produce pure stevioside or rebaudioside A. Rebaudioside A is also known as rebiana, and is sold under the trade names Truvia™ and PureVia™. Stevioside has the European Registry Number E960.

How does it taste?

Dried stevia leaves are sweet, with a potency of about 30 times sucrose on a weight basis. Unfortunately, there is some bitterness and a licorice-like taste associated with stevia sweeteners. Pure stevioside has a sweetness potency of about 210 times sucrose on a weight basis, with measurable bitterness and licorice-like taste. Rebaudioside A has a sweetness potency of about 200 times sucrose. It has less bitterness, but retains the licorice-like taste. Stevia sweeteners also differ from sucrose in their temporal (time-intensity) profiles. Sweetness starts slowly, and it lingers in the mouth longer than sucrose.

How well does it work?

Stevioside and rebaudioside are stable indefinitely in the dry state. They are also stable under most conditions in food products. Even under baking conditions, the stability is very good except in high acid products (pH 3 or lower).

How many calories?

Stevioside and rebaudioside are composed of steviol with two or more sugars attached. In the digestive system, bacteria remove the sugars, leaving free steviol. Because of the high potency of stevia sweeteners, the amount of sweetener used is very small, so the amount of sugar produced is not significant in terms of calorie intake. Stevia-based sweeteners are essentially zero calorie products. Their glycemic index is 0.

Is it safe?

Stevia sweeteners are attractive to consumers because they are natural (although it's useful to remember that "natural" is not the same as "safe"). Stevia has been consumed in South America for hundreds of years, and in Japan for over 30 years, providing some empirical evidence of safety.

Stevia glycosides do not support the growth of microorganisms that cause dental caries.

Carefully controlled animal studies have generally shown no effects. The exception is that, at high levels in the diet, animals consume less food and lose weight, probably due to the presence of bitter taste, but this only occurs when the sweetener makes up 5% or more of the diet. Studies in humans have looked for effects on blood pressure, blood glucose, and have generally found no effect. Animal studies have also looked for effects on fetal development, and none have been found.

In the digestive system, bacteria remove the sugars, leaving free steviol. Free steviol is absorbed by the body and metabolized to a glucuronide (in the liver, glucuronic acid is attached to the steviol, making it more water-soluble so that it can be excreted in the urine or bile).

The toxicity of free steviol has been controversial. Steviol showed mutagenic activity in some bacteria-based tests, but not in others. More sophisticated tests, using human blood cells, show no mutagenic activity. Furthermore, conversion of steviol to the glucuronide appears to be so rapid that free steviol cannot be detected in humans, even with extremely sensitive detection methods.

Overall, the safety studies indicate that stevia based sweeteners are safe for human use. Japan approved the use of stevia sweeteners in the 1970s. Brazil, China, Korea, Paraguay, and more recently, Australia and New Zealand have also approved their use. In December 2008, the FDA issued a "no objection" notification for rebiana meaning that it is now "generally recognized as safe."

Luo han guo

What is it?

Luo han guo (also known as luo han kuo and as monk fruit) is the fruit of *Siraitia grosvenorii*, a vine that grows in southern China and other parts of southeast Asia. The sweetness of the fruit comes partly from sugars, and partly from a series of triterpene glycosides called "mogrosides."

Nectresse™ is a blend of luo han guo extract, erythritol, sucrose, and molasses.

How does it taste?

The mogrosides are up to 300 times as sweet as sucrose, and they have a slight licorice-like off taste.

How well does it work?

Mogrosides have good water solubility and heat stability.

How many calories?

The mogrosides do not contribute any calories to the diet. Of course, if you were to consume the fruit, with its sugars, there would be calories and an effect on blood glucose. In the luo han guo based product Nectresse™, each packet has small amounts of sugar, molasses, and erythritol, but these contribute less than 5 calories per packet, so the FDA allows it to be labeled "no calorie." The mogrosides have a glycemic index of 0.

Is it safe?

Luo han guo has been cultivated and consumed for centuries in Asia. It has GRAS status in the United States, but does not yet have regulatory approval in Europe.

The mogrosides do not support the growth of microorganisms that cause dental caries. Luo han guo extracts that include fruit sugars could do so.

Glycyrrhizin

What is it?

Glycyrrhizin (also known as glycyrrhizic acid) is a triterpenoid saponin that comes from the root of licorice, *Glycyhrrhiza glabra*. It is usually extracted as a potassium, calcium, or ammonium salt. The plant is native to Turkey, Iraq, Spain, Greece, and northern China. Glycyrrhizin has the European Registry Number E958.

How does it taste?

Glycyrrhizin has a sweet taste with a characteristic licorice taste sometimes described as "cooling." The potency is about 50 times that of sucrose. The sweetness is slow in onset and tends to linger.

How well does it work?

Because of its slow onset, characteristic licorice-like taste, and mouth cooling property, glycyrrhizin is not often used as the sole sweetener in foods or beverages.

How many calories?

Glycyrrhizin provides little or no caloric value. It has a glycemic index of 0.

Is it safe?

Glycyrrhizin (as a component of licorice root) has a long history of use as a sweetener and as an herbal remedy. Studies have demonstrated that glycyrrhizin inhibits an enzyme that normally inactivates cortisol, so that consumption of licorice or glycyrrhizin in excess can raise the level of cortisol in the body above normal levels. Cortisol has anti-inflammatory properties, so glycyrrhizin can be beneficial in treating some conditions, but excessive cortisol can cause water retention, hypertension, and loss of potassium and calcium.

Glycyrrhizin has GRAS status in the United States for use as a flavoring agent, but not for use as a sweetener. The European Union's Scientific Committee on Food recommended an upper limit of 100 mg/day, which corresponds to about two ounces per day of licorice candy. The Food and Drug Administration stated that, for persons over 40 years of age, eating two ounces of black licorice a day for two weeks could cause serious health problems. A similar limit is recommended in Japan. Excess cortisol during pregnancy correlates with low birth weight, so glycyrrhizin and licorice consumption are discouraged during pregnancy.

Glycyrrhizin does not support the growth of microorganisms that cause dental caries.

Thaumatin

What is it?

The katemfe plant (*Thaumatococcus daniellii* Benth, also called "the miraculous fruit of the Sudan") is common in the West African rain forest zone. The fruit contains 1-3 black seeds surrounded by a gel, and capped with a membranous sac, the aril, which has a sweet taste. This is used as a sweetener in cooking, in flavoring palm wine, and in making confections for children.

Thaumatin is a protein which is isolated from the katemfe fruit. Thaumatin has the European Registry Number E957.

How does it taste?

Thaumatin is sweet, with a slow onset, lingering sweetness and a licorice after-taste. Thaumatin is about 2000 times as sweet as sucrose, on a weight basis.

How well does it work?

Thaumatin has good stability to heat. Because of its slow onset and licorice off-taste, thaumatin is not routinely used as a sweetener.

How many calories?

Since thaumatin is a protein, it provides 4 calories per gram. However, its high potency means that very little would be needed to provide a high level of sweetness, so the actual number of calories that would be added would be 1 or less. Thaumatin has a glycemic index of 0.

Is it safe?

Thaumatin is digested like any other protein, so there is no concern about toxicity. Thaumatin has been tested for toxicity, digestibility, teratogenicity, and allergenicity. It is non-toxic, it is readily digested, and it is not teratogenic. It is allergenic, but less so than house dust mites.

In the United States, the Food and Drug Administration has classified thaumatin as GRAS for use as a flavor enhancer, with FEMA GRAS Number 3732. Thaumatin was approved by JECFA in 1985. In Europe it was approved in 1988 as a sweetener and flavor enhancer.

Thaumatin does not support the growth of microorganisms that cause dental caries.

Brazzein

What is it?

Brazzein is a small protein produced by the fruit of a West African plant, *Pentadiplandra brazzeana* Baillon. The fruit is consumed by the people of Gabon and Cameroon.

How does it taste?

Brazzein is sweet, with a slow onset, lingering sweetness and some licorice after-taste. Brazzein is about 1000 times as sweet as sucrose, on a weight basis.

How well does it work?

Brazzein has good stability to heat. It is not yet marketed as a commercial product or ingredient in the United States. Because of its slow onset and licorice off-taste, brazzein is not likely to be used as a sole sweetener for foods and beverages.

How many calories?

Since brazzein is a protein, it provides 4 calories per gram. However, its high potency means that very little would be needed to provide a high level of sweetness, so the actual number of calories that would be added would be 1 or less. Brazzein has a glycemic index of 0.

Is it safe?

Brazzein is digested like any other protein, so there is no concern about toxicity. In the United States, a producer of brazzein (Natur Research Ingredients) has self-affirmed brazzein as GRAS.

Brazzein does not support the growth of microorganisms that cause dental caries.

Monellin

What is it?

Monellin is a protein produced by the fruit of a West African plant called "serendipity berry" (*Dioscoreophyllum cumminsii*).

How does it taste?

Monellin is about 2,000 times as sweet as sucrose. Like all of the protein sweeteners, it has a slow onset and lingering sweet aftertaste.

How well does it work?

Monellin does not have good heat stability. Its slow onset and lingering aftertaste limit its usefulness as a sweetener.

How many calories?

Since monellin is a protein, it provides 4 calories per gram. However, its high potency means that very little would be needed to provide a high level of sweetness, so the actual number of calories that would be added to a food or beverage would be 1 or less. Monellin has a glycemic index of 0.

Is it safe?

Monellin has no regulatory approval in the United States or Europe. This is because it is difficult to produce in quantity, has poor stability, and has limitations in its taste quality. Since it is a protein, it is expected to have no safety issues. It has been consumed for centuries in Africa.

Monellin does not support the growth of microorganisms that cause dental caries.

Mabinlin

What is it?

The mabinlins are a family of proteins extracted from the seeds of mabinlang (*Capparis masaikai* Levl.), a plant that grows in Yunnan province of China. The fruit is about the size of a tennis ball. The proteins are named mabinlin-1, -2, -3, and -4. Mabinlin-2 is the sweetest and best characterized of these proteins.

How does it taste?

Mabinlin-2 is about 100 times as sweet as sucrose on a weight basis. Like all of the protein sweeteners, it has a slow onset and lingering sweet aftertaste.

How well does it work?

Mabinlin-2 has good heat stability. Its slow onset and lingering aftertaste limit its usefulness as a sweetener.

How many calories?

Since mabinlin is a protein, it provides 4 calories per gram. Its higher potency relative to sucrose means that it could provide significant calorie reduction when used as a sucrose replacement. Mabinlin has a glycemic index of 0.

Is it safe?

Mabinlin has no regulatory approval in the United States or Europe. Since it is a protein, it is expected to have no safety issues. It has been consumed for centuries in China.

Mabinlin does not support the growth of microorganisms that cause dental caries.

Curculin

What is it?

Curculin is a protein isolated from a fruit called lumbah or lemba (*Curculigo latifolia*), a plant that grows in Malaysia.

How does it taste?

Curculin is about 1000 times as sweet as sucrose on a weight basis. Like all of the protein sweeteners, it has a slow onset and lingering sweet aftertaste. Curculin also has a taste modifying property similar to miraculin (described below). After curculin is consumed, it causes water and sour solutions to taste sweet. This effect lasts for 5-10 minutes.

How well does it work?

Curculin has poor heat stability. Its slow onset and lingering aftertaste limit its usefulness as a sweetener.

How many calories?

Since curculin is a protein, it provides 4 calories per gram. Its higher potency relative to sucrose means that it could provide significant calorie reduction when used as a sucrose replacement. Curculin has a glycemic index of 0.

Is it safe?

Curculin has no regulatory approval in the United States or Europe. Since it is a protein, it is expected to have no safety issues. It has been consumed for centuries in Malaysia.

Curculin does not support the growth of microorganisms that cause dental caries.

Miraculin

What is it?
Miraculin is a protein isolated from a fruit called "miracle fruit" or
"miracle berry" (*Synsepalum dulcificum*), a plant that grows in West
Africa.

How does it taste?
Miraculin does not taste sweet. However, after miraculin is consumed,
it causes sour solutions to taste sweet. This effect lasts for up to an hour.

How well does it work?
Miraculin's usefulness as a sweetener is limited by the need to pretreat
the tongue, in order to produce sweetness, as well as the long duration
of the effect.

How many calories?
Since miraculin is a protein, it provides 4 calories per gram. Only
small quantities are needed to produce sweetness, so it could provide
significant calorie reduction if used as a sucrose replacement. Miraculin
has a glycemic index of 0.

Is it safe?
Miraculin has no regulatory approval in the United States. It reportedly
has novel food status in Europe, and it is approved as a harmless
additive in Japan. Since it is a protein, it is expected to have no safety
issues. It has been consumed for centuries in West Africa.

Miraculin does not support the growth of microorganisms that cause
dental caries.

Historic Sweeteners

As I discussed earlier, everything is toxic, depending on the dose. Historically, a number of different sweet tasting substances have been used, and have later been found to be unacceptable for safety reasons. Here are a few examples.

Lead acetate

Lead (II) acetate is also known as sugar of lead, because it is a white crystalline substance and it has a sweet taste. Lead has been known to be toxic for a very long time. However, lead acetate has periodically been found as an adulterant in foods and beverages.

Dulcin

Dulcin was discovered in 1884, about 6 years after saccharin, and it lacks saccharin's bitter aftertaste. Early safety studies in dogs and rabbits gave mixed results. Dulcin was used until 1951, when an FDA study led to its removal from the market.

Glucin

Glucin was a substance described as "amido-triazin-sulfonic acid." Its exact structure is not known, but it is thought to be similar to saccharin. It was used for a period of time in the first half of the 20th century. It was banned by the FDA because of health concerns.

P-4000

In 1940, a Dutch chemist named J.J. Blanksma discovered a series of sweet-tasting nitroanilines. One of these, P-4000, derived its name from the fact that it is 4,000 times as sweet as sucrose. During World War II, P-4000 was used as a sweetener in the Netherlands and Berlin because of sugar shortages. It has been marketed as "Ultrasüss." Nitroanilines are now known, as a group, to be fairly toxic. P-4000 was banned by the FDA in 1950.

Tales of Sweetener Discovery

I really enjoy the stories about how various sweeteners were discovered. Almost all of them were discovered accidentally. Here, I want to share some of these stories with you.

Saccharin

There is some controversy over the discovery of saccharin. Constantine Fahlberg was working in the laboratory of Ira Remsen at Johns Hopkins University in 1879. According to Fahlberg's account, he accidentally spilled some laboratory material on his hand, and noticed the sweet taste later in the evening when he was eating dinner. Fahlberg and Remsen published the work jointly. Later Fahlberg patented saccharin without including Remsen on the patent. Fahlberg went on to become wealthy. Remsen went on to become the president of Johns Hopkins University, and he commented "Fahlberg is a scoundrel. It nauseates me to hear my name mentioned in the same breath with him."

Cyclamate

Michael Sveda was a graduate student at the University of Illinois, working in the laboratory of L.F. Audrieth on the synthesis of anti-pyretic (anti-fever) drugs. While working in the laboratory in 1937, he put his cigarette down on the lab bench. When he put it back in his mouth, he discovered the sweet taste of cyclamate.

Aspartame

It was December, 1965. Jim Schlatter, a chemist at G.D. Searle, was working on a project to discover new treatments for gastric ulcers. To test new anti-ulcer drugs, the biologists used a tetrapeptide (four amino acids) normally produced in the stomach. Schlatter was synthesizing this tetrapeptide in the lab, and one of the steps in the process was to make a dipeptide intermediate, aspartyl-phenylalanine methyl ester.

In the course of his work, Schlatter accidentally got a small amount of the compound on his hands without noticing it. Later that morning, he licked his finger as he reached for a piece of paper, and noticed a sweet taste. His curiosity drove him to ask "Where did that sweet taste come from?" His first thought was of the doughnut he had eaten during his coffee break, but he realized that he had been to the bathroom and had washed his hands since then. It could only be the aspartyl-phenylalanine methyl ester he had worked with. He knew that aspartic acid and phenylalanine, which make up this product, are natural amino acids present in all proteins, so he felt it would be safe to taste the material.

It was sweet! He and his lab partner, Harman Lowrie, both tasted the material in 10 milliliters of black coffee, noting the sweet taste as well as the absence of any bitter aftertaste, and recorded the results in Schlatter's laboratory notebook. His boss, Robert Mazur, convinced the company of the potential value of this discovery. Twenty years later, Schlatter's curiosity had produced a billion dollar per year sweetener.

Acesulfame

Acesulfame was discovered by a chemist, Karl Clauss, in 1967. He was synthesizing a new class of heterocyclic chemicals in the laboratory. He noticed a sweet taste when he licked his finger to pick up a piece of paper.

Sucralose

Sucralose may have the strangest "accidental discovery" story of all the sweeteners. Tate & Lyle, a British sugar company, was looking for ways to use sucrose as a chemical intermediate. In collaboration with Prof. Leslie Hough's laboratory at King's College in London, halogenated sugars were being synthesized and tested. In 1976, a foreign graduate student, Shashikant Phadnis, misunderstood a request for "testing" of a chlorinated sugar as a request for "tasting," leading to the discovery that many chlorinated sugars are sweet, with potencies some hundreds or thousands of times as great as sucrose.

Conclusion

Which sweetener is best?

For me, this is the most frequent of frequently asked questions. The answer depends on several factors, which you have to prioritize for yourself. If taste quality is your top criterion, you should stick to sugars (sucrose or high fructose corn syrup, for example). If calories are your main concern, you may want a sugar alcohol (sorbitol, lactitol, xylitol), a high potency sweetener (aspartame, saccharin, sucralose) or one of the natural product sweeteners (stevia, luo han guo). However, each of these has its own drawbacks that must be considered. If safety is at the top of your list, you can use any sweetener, as long as you do so in moderation. If "natural" is your first consideration, you may wish to focus on the sugars and natural products. But remember that "natural" is not the same as "harmless." Sorbitol and glycyrrhizin are both natural, but they both have the potential to cause harm.

The second most frequently asked question is "What do you use?" I usually use sugar, with a great deal of moderation. I don't often use other sweeteners, but when I do, I prefer aspartame. The taste quality is quite good, and I know exactly how my body will deal with it.

References

1. Schiffman SS, Buckley CE, Sampson HA, Massey EW, Baraniuk JN, Follett JV, Warwick ZS. Aspartame and susceptibility to headache. N Engl J Med 1987; 317:1181-1185.

2. Rulis AM, Levitt JA. FDA's food ingredient approval process. Regul Toxicol Pharmacol 2009; 53(1):20-31; http://www.caloriecontrol.org/pdf/Rulis_08.pdf.

3. Atkinson FS, Foster-Powell K, Brand-Miller JC. International Tables of Glycemic Index and Glycemic Load Values: 2008. Diab Care 2008; 31(12).

4. Fitch C, Keim KS. Position of the Academy of Nutrition and Dietetics: Use of Nutritive and Nonnutritive Sweeteners. J Acad Nutr Diet 2012; 112:739-758.

5. Milgrom P, Ly KA, Rothen M. Xylitol and its vehicles for public health needs. Adv Dent Res 2009; 21:44-47.

6. Storey D et al. Gastrointestinal tolerance of erythritol and xylitol ingested in a liquid. Eur J Clin Nutr 2007; 61:349-354.

7. Whysner J, Williams GM. Saccharin mechanistic data and risk assessment: urine composition, enhanced cell proliferation, and tumor promotion. Pharmacol Ther 1996; 71:225-252.

Index

Appendices

Abbreviations and acronyms

The following abbreviations and acronyms are used in this book.

Abbreviation	Meaning
ADI	Acceptable Daily Intake
EFSA	European Food Safety Authority, an agency of the European Union
FDA	United Stated Food and Drug Administration
FEMA	Flavor and Extract Manufacturers Association
GI	Glycemic Index
GL	Glycemic Load
GRAS	Generally Recognized As Safe
HFCS	High Fructose Corn Syrup
IOM	Institute of Medicine
JECFA	Joint FAO/WHO Expert Committee on Food Additives. FAO is the Food and Agriculture Organization of the United Nations, and WHO is the World Health Organization, another United Nations Agency
LTV	Laxative threshold value
NOAEL	No Observable Adverse Effect Level
RDI	Recommended daily intake

Acceptable Daily Intake (ADI) data, in milligrams per kilogram of body weight per day, except as noted.

Sweetener	FDA	JECFA	EFSA
Acesulfame K	15	15	9
Alitame	Not approved	1	
Aspartame	50	40	40
Cyclamate	Not approved	11	7
Glycyrrhizin	GRAS. Recommended limit of 2 ounces black licorice per day		Recommended upper limit of 100 milligrams per day
Neohesperidin DHC	GRAS as flavor enhancer. Not approved as sweetener	not evaluated	5
Neotame	18 mg/day	2	2
Saccharin	5	5	5
Stevia (as steviol)	GRAS	4 (equivalent to 12 for rebaudioside A)	4 (equivalent to 12 for rebaudioside A)
Sucralose	5	15	15
Thaumatin	GRAS as flavor enhancer. Not approved as sweetener	Not specified	Acceptable

Glycemic Index (GI) for sweeteners, based on glucose = 100

Sweetener	Glycemic Index	Reference
Sucrose	65	1
Brown sugar	65	
Molasses	55	
Fructose	15	1
Glucose	103	1
Lactose	46	1
Isomaltulose	32 (calculated)	2
Corn syrup	100	
High fructose corn syrup	55 (calculated)	3
Honey	35-87, depending on sugars 61 (average)	1
Agave syrup	13	1
Sorbitol	9	4
Isomalt	9	4
Lactitol	6	4
Maltitol	35	4
Mannitol	0	4
Xylitol	13	4
Tagatose	3	5
Erythritol	0	4
Glycerol	0	6
Acesulfame	0	7
Aspartame	0	7
Cyclamate	0	7
Neohesperidin dihydrochalcone	0	7
Neotame	0	7
Saccharin	0	7
Sucralose	0	7
Alitame	0	7
Stevioside, rebaudiosides	0	7
Mogrosides	0	7
Glycyrrhizin	0	7
Thaumatin	0	7
Brazzein	0	7
Monellin	0	7
Mabinlin	0	7
Curculin	0	7
Miraculin	0	7

1. Atkinson FS, Foster-Powell K, Brand-Miller JC. International Tables of Glycemic Index and Glycemic Load Values: 2008. Diab Care 2008; 31(12).

2. Holub I, Gostner A, Theis S, Nosek L, Kudlich T, Melcher R, Scheppach W. Novel findings on the metabolic effects of the low glycaemic carbohydrate isomaltulose (Palatinose™). Br J Nutr 2010; 103(12):1730-1737.

3. Calculated from fructose and glucose values, for HFCS containing 55% fructose, 45% glucose.

4. Livesey G. Health potential of polyols as sugar replacers, with emphasis on low glycaemic properties. Nutr Res Rev 2003; 16:163-191.

5. Sydney University's Glycemic Index Research Service (Human Nutrition Unit, University of Sydney, Australia), www.glycemicindex. com, accessed 17 January 2013.

6. Wolever TMS. Oral glycerin has a negligible effect on plasma glucose and insulin in normal subjects. Diabetes 2005; 51(Suppl 2):A602.

7. Glycemic index is not measured for high potency sweeteners, because it is understood that (a) glycemic index is based on carbohydrate content, and most high potency sweeteners do not contain carbohydrate, and (b) most high potency sweeteners cannot produce glucose, and (c) their use level is so low that any glucose produced would be negligible. I list a GI value of 0 for these sweeteners, but these values are not based on actual experimentation. It would be unpleasant and impractical to ask a human being to consume 25 or 50 grams of any of these substances, and the resulting number would be meaningless.

E numbers (assigned by the European Union)

E number	Sweetener
E420	Sorbitol
E421	Mannitol
E422	Glycerol
E950	Acesulfame K
E951	Aspartame
E952	Cyclamate
E953	Isomalt
E954	Saccharin
E955	Sucralose
E956	Alitame
E957	Thaumatin
E958	Glycyrrhizin
E959	Neohesperidin dihydrochalcone
E960	Steviol glycosides
E961	Neotame
E962	Aspartame + acesulfame salt
E965	Maltitol
E966	Lactitol
E967	Xylitol
E968	Erythritol

Made in the USA
Lexington, KY
21 March 2017